HOW CAN HEALTH CARE ORGANIZATIONS BECOME MORE HEALTH LITERATE?

WORKSHOP SUMMARY

Lyla M. Hernandez, *Rapporteur*

Roundtable on Health Literacy

Board on Population Health and Public Health Practice

INSTITUTE OF MEDICINE
OF THE NATIONAL ACADEMIES

THE NATIONAL ACADEMIES PRESS
Washington, D.C.
www.nap.edu

THE NATIONAL ACADEMIES PRESS 500 Fifth Street, NW Washington, DC 20001

NOTICE: The project that is the subject of this report was approved by the Governing Board of the National Research Council, whose members are drawn from the councils of the National Academy of Sciences, the National Academy of Engineering, and the Institute of Medicine.

This study was supported by contracts between the National Academy of Sciences and Aetna, the Agency for Healthcare Research and Quality (HHSP233200900537P), the American College of Physicians, America's Health Insurance Plans, GlaxoSmithKline, the Health Resources and Services Administration (HHSH25034004T), Johnson & Johnson, the East Bay Foundation (Kaiser Permanente), Merck and Co., Inc., and the Missouri Foundation for Health (09-0290-HL-09). Any opinions, findings, conclusions, or recommendations expressed in this publication are those of the author(s) and do not necessarily reflect the view of the organizations or agencies that provided support for this project.

International Standard Book Number-13: 978-0-309-25681-0
International Standard Book Number-10: 0-309-25681-X

Additional copies of this report are available from the National Academies Press, 500 Fifth Street, NW, Keck 360, Washington, DC 20001; (800) 624-6242 or (202) 334-3313; http://www.nap.edu.

For more information about the Institute of Medicine, visit the IOM home page at: www.iom.edu.

Printed in the United States of America

The serpent has been a symbol of long life, healing, and knowledge among almost all cultures and religions since the beginning of recorded history. The serpent adopted as a logotype by the Institute of Medicine is a relief carving from ancient Greece, now held by the Staatliche Museen in Berlin.

Suggested citation: IOM (Institute of Medicine). 2012. *How Can Health Care Organizations Become More Health Literate?: Workshop Summary*. Washington, DC: The National Academies Press.

*"Knowing is not enough; we must apply.
Willing is not enough; we must do."*
—Goethe

INSTITUTE OF MEDICINE
OF THE NATIONAL ACADEMIES

Advising the Nation. Improving Health.

PLANNING COMMITTEE ON ATTRIBUTES OF A HEALTH LITERATE ORGANIZATION[1]

CYNTHIA BAUR, Senior Advisor for Health Literacy, Office of the Associate Director for Communication, Centers for Disease Control and Prevention, U.S. Department of Health and Human Services

CINDY BRACH, Senior Health Policy Researcher, Center for Delivery, Organization, and Markets, Agency for Healthcare Research and Quality, U.S. Department of Health and Human Services

BENARD DREYER, Professor of Pediatrics, New York University, NYU Langone Medical Center, New York

JEAN KRAUSE, Executive Vice President and Chief Executive Officer, American College of Physicians Foundation

RUTH PARKER, Professor of Medicine, Emory University School of Medicine

PAUL SCHYVE, Senior Advisor, Quality Improvement, The Joint Commission

[1] Institute of Medicine planning committees are solely responsible for organizing the workshop, identifying topics, and choosing speakers. The responsibility for the published workshop summary rests with the workshop rapporteur and the institution.

ROUNDTABLE ON HEALTH LITERACY[1]

[1] Institute of Medicine forums and roundtables do not issue, review, or approve individual documents. The responsibility for the published workshop summary rests with the workshop rapporteur and the institution.

ANDREW PLEASANT, Health Literacy and Research Director, Canyon Ranch Institute
SCOTT C. RATZAN, Vice President, Global Health, Johnson & Johnson
WILL ROSS, Associate Dean for Diversity, Associate Professor of Medicine, Washington University School of Medicine
PAUL M. SCHYVE, Senior Vice President, The Joint Commission
PATRICK WAYTE, Vice President, Marketing and Health Education, American Heart Association
WINSTON F. WONG, Medical Director, Community Benefit, Disparities Improvement and Quality Initiatives, Kaiser Permanente

Study Staff

LYLA M. HERNANDEZ, Roundtable Director
ANDREW LEMERISE, Research Associate
ANGELA MARTIN, Senior Program Assistant
ROSE MARIE MARTINEZ, Director, Board on Population Health and Public Health Practice

Reviewers

This report has been reviewed in draft form by individuals chosen for their diverse perspectives and technical expertise, in accordance with procedures approved by the National Research Council's Report Review Committee. The purpose of this independent review is to provide candid and critical comments that will assist the institution in making its published report as sound as possible and to ensure that the report meets institutional standards for objectivity, evidence, and responsiveness to the study charge. The review comments and draft manuscript remain confidential to protect the integrity of the process. We wish to thank the following individuals for their review of this report:

Cynthia Baur, Centers for Disease Control and Prevention
Yolanda Partida, University of California, San Francisco
Lee Sanders, Stanford University
Sarah Hudson Scholle, National Committee for Quality Assurance

Although the reviewers listed above have provided many constructive comments and suggestions, they did not see the final draft of the report before its release. The review of this report was overseen by **Harold Fallon,** University of South Carolina. Appointed by the Institute of Medicine, he was responsible for making certain that an independent examination of this report was carried out in accordance with institutional procedures and that all review comments were carefully considered. Responsibility for the final content of this report rests entirely with the rapporteur and the institution.

Acknowledgments

The sponsors of the Institute of Medicine Roundtable on Health Literacy made it possible to plan and conduct the workshop Attributes of a Health Literate Organization. Sponsors from the U.S. Department of Health and Human Services are the Agency for Healthcare Research and Quality and the Health Resources and Services Administration. Nonfederal sponsorship was provided by Aetna; the American College of Physicians Foundation; the American Health Insurance Plans; the East Bay Community Foundation (Kaiser Permanente); GlaxoSmithKline; Johnson & Johnson; Merck and Co., Inc.; and the Missouri Foundation for Health.

The Roundtable wishes to extend its appreciation to Dean Schillinger and Debra Keller for their excellent paper exploring the attributes of a health literate organization. The roundtable also wishes to express its gratitude to the following speakers for their thoughtful and stimulating presentations: William R. Calnon, Debra Dever, Cynthia Horton, Isabel V. Hoverman, Debra Keller, Shari M. Ling, John Neuberger, Ana Pujols-McKee, Dean Schillinger, Darren Townzen, and Ross Wilson. The planning committee members are to be commended for their work in developing an excellent workshop agenda. Members of the planning committee were Cynthia Baur, Cindy Brach, Benard Dreyer, Jean Krause, Ruth Parker, and Paul Schyve.

Contents

BOXES

FIGURES

1

Introduction[1]

Health literacy is the degree to which individuals have the capacity to obtain, process, and understand basic health information and services needed to make appropriate health care decisions (IOM, 2004).

Low health literacy is a significant problem in the United States, with more than 36 percent of the adult population (approximately 80 million people) having poor health literacy (AHRQ, 2011). While a lack of health literacy is more likely to be an issue with more vulnerable populations, the problem affects all social and demographic groups. Some of the difficulties experienced by individuals with limited health literacy include problems in communicating with clinicians, greater barriers in managing chronic illness, less likelihood of receiving preventive care, a greater likelihood of experiencing serious medication errors, increased risk of hospitalization, and poorer quality of life (AHRQ, 2011).

The Institute of Medicine (IOM) Roundtable on Health Literacy focuses on bringing together leaders from the federal government, foundations, health plans, associations, and private companies to address challenges facing health literacy practice and research and to identify approaches to promote health literacy in both the public and private sectors. The roundtable serves to educate the public, press, and policy makers regarding the issues of health literacy, sponsoring workshops to

[1] This workshop was organized by an independent planning committee whose role was limited to identification of topics and speakers. This workshop summary was prepared by the rapporteur as a factual summary of the presentations and discussions that took place at the workshop. Statements, recommendations, and opinions expressed are those of individual presenters and participants, and are not necessarily endorsed or verified by the Roundtable or the National Academies, and they should not be construed as reflecting any group consensus.

discuss approaches to resolve health literacy challenges. It also builds partnerships to move the field of health literacy forward by translating research findings into practical strategies for implementation.

Most health literacy research has focused on patient skills and abilities and on interventions designed to improve those skills and abilities. However, there is growing recognition that health literacy depends not only on individual skills and abilities but also on the demands and complexities of the health care system. It is of primary importance therefore, to develop strategies that health care organizations can use to improve their health literacy–promoting attributes. Yet organizations often find it difficult to determine exactly what it means to be health literate.

The roundtable decided to commission a paper that would present and explore a set of attributes that define a health literate health care organization. A health literate health care organization is defined as "an organization that makes it easier for people to navigate, understand, and use information and services to take care of their health" (Brach et al., 2012). Developing such a paper was a tremendous challenge, and the roundtable is very appreciative that Dr. Dean Schillinger, with the assistance of Dr. Debra Keller, consented to write the paper. The focus of the workshop was to unveil the paper and to receive feedback and input on the ideas presented. Based on the feedback from the workshop as well as from other sources, the paper on attributes will be revised.

The workshop was organized by an independent planning committee in accordance with the procedures of the National Academy of Sciences. The planning group was composed of Cynthia Baur, Cindy Brach, Benard Dreyer, Jean Krause, Ruth Parker, and Paul Schyve. The workshop featured the presentation of a commissioned paper on the attributes of a health literate organization and invited presentations and discussions in reaction to the paper as well as discussion of other topics related to health literacy. The workshop was moderated by roundtable chair, George Isham, and featured presentations and discussions. Chapter 2 is the presentation of the commissioned paper. Chapters 3, 4, and 5 describe the reactions of providers from different health care settings, including a health care executive working in a public hospital system, the director of a public clinic, a physician in private practice, a pharmacist in a pharmacy chain, a dentist in private practice, and a nurse from a visiting nurses association. This workshop summary report is not meant to imply that the presenters' views can be generalized as representative of the opinions of all providers in a particular type of health care setting. Rather, the report is a summary of the presentations made. Each of these individuals was asked to address the following questions:

1. Which attributes would be your top priorities?
2. Is your organization likely to undertake activities to implement these attributes?
3. What are the challenges to implementing those attributes?
4. Which attributes do you feel you are already making progress on?
5. What incentives would make your organization more likely to take on this work?
6. Are there any attributes you think are infeasible or undesirable? Why?

Chapter 6 summarizes the presentations of the final workshop panel, which consisted of speakers from organizations that can or do provide incentives for other organizations to engage in specific activities such as implementing health literacy approaches. These presenters were asked to address the following questions:

1. Which attributes do you think are most important? Why?
2. Are there any attributes you think unfeasible or undesirable? Which ones and why?
3. What do you think are the challenges for implementing these attributes?
4. How could your organization encourage the implementation of these attributes?

Chapter 7, the final chapter, includes a general discussion of the workshop's presentations.

REFERENCES

AHRQ (Agency for Healthcare Research and Quality). 2011. Health Literacy Interventions and Outcomes: An Updated Systematic Review. Evidence Report/Technology Assessment, No. 199. http://www.ahrq.gov/clinic/epcsums/litupsum.htm (accessed December 10, 2011).

Brach C., B. Deyer, P. Schyve, L. M. Hernandez, C. Bauer, A. J. Lemerise, and R. Parker. 2012. *Attributes of a Health Literate Organization*. Discussion Paper, Institute of Medicine, Washington, DC. www.iom.edu/healthlit10attributes (accessed April 4, 2012).

IOM (Institute of Medicine). 2004. *Health literacy: A prescription to end confusion*. Washington, DC: The National Academies Press.

2

Attributes of a Health Literate Health Care Organization

THE OTHER SIDE OF THE COIN: ATTRIBUTES OF A HEALTH LITERATE HEALTH CARE ORGANIZATION

Dean Schillinger, M.D.
Debra Keller, M.D., M.P.H.
University of California, San Francisco

Most health literacy research, Schillinger said, has focused on characterizing patients' deficits, on how best to measure a patient's health literacy, and on clarifying the relationships between limited health literacy and health outcomes. There is now a growing appreciation that health literacy represents a balance between an individual's health literacy and the health literacy demands and attributes of the health care system. The commissioned paper (see Appendix A) discussed in this presentation is an attempt to advance a conversation about the health care organization side of the health literacy dynamic.

There is increasing interest from multiple stakeholders in addressing the system level factors that contribute to the high literacy demands of the health care system. Implementation of the Patient Protection and Affordable Care Act (ACA)[1] provides both opportunities and challenges, especially for individuals with limited literacy, whether it is with respect

[1] A summary of the ACA can be found at http://dpc.senate.gov/healthreformbill/healthbill04.pdf (accessed February 6, 2012).

to insurance reform, accessing and taking advantage of Medicaid expansion, maximizing one's experience in a patient-centered medical home, or benefiting from the diffusion of information technology into health care.

This paper attempts to identify and describe a set of attributes for health care organizations that will enable these organizations to mitigate the negative consequences of limited health literacy and to improve access to and the quality, safety, and value of health care services. The attributes identified in this paper are not intended to describe a specific type of organization; rather it is the case that organizations aspiring to these attributes are those that are committed to implementing improvements. They are organizations committed to reengineering systems in order to better accommodate the communication needs of populations with limited health literacy, that is, to become health literate health care organizations.

The paper is most applicable to organizations that provide direct care to patients. However, the paper also attempts to be relevant to the broader range of organizations and institutions that comprise the very complex and modern U.S. health care system. Organizational investments are needed to maximize patients' and families' capacities (see Box 2-1) in a number of areas.

The framework for the attributes of a health literate health care organization can be represented by a pyramid (Figure 2-1). The attributes fall into one or more of the rows of the pyramid. At the base of the pyramid is organizational commitment. The second tier is an accessible educational technology infrastructure. The third row of the pyramid is an augmented workforce. The fourth row is embedded policies and practices, and at the top of the pyramid is effective bidirectional communication.

The structure of this pyramid follows a clear logic. The foundation of becoming a health literate organization is organizational commitment. This is followed by infrastructure, followed by a well-trained workforce, followed by policies and procedures that the workforce and the infrastructure can support so that, in the end, effective bidirectional communication can take place.

Attributes

This paper presents 18 attributes health care organizations that wish to be health literate should strive for (see Box 2-2). It is important to note that it is not expected that any organization currently possesses all of these attributes. Rather, the paper is an attempt to offer a vision of how organizations should evolve in order to become more responsive to the needs of populations with limited health literacy, thereby improving care for all.

BOX 2-1
Patient and Family Capacities to Maximize

Ability to

- comprehend and engage in preventive health behaviors and to receive preventive health care services if desired;
- recognize changes in their health states that require attention and then access health care services appropriately;
- develop meaningful ongoing relationships with health care providers that are based on open communication and trust;
- obtain timely and accurate diagnoses for both acute and chronic health conditions; comprehend the meaning of their illness, the options for treatment, and anticipated health outcomes;
- build and refine skills needed to safely and effectively manage these conditions at home and communicate with the health care team when the illness trajectory changes;
- report their communication needs or comprehension gaps;
- make informed health care decisions that reflect their wishes and their values;
- navigate transitions in care; and
- make health care coverage choices based on their families' health needs, better comprehend the range of benefits and services available to them and how to access those services, and be more aware of the financial implications of health care choices in order to improve decision making.

ATTRIBUTE 1: Health literate health care organizations promote health literacy as an organizational responsibility. This implies that such organizations promote a culture of clear communication and make such communication an organizational priority. They raise organization-wide awareness of the importance of health literacy and take responsibility for effective communication. They build health literacy concerns into their organizational operations, strategic planning, job descriptions, evaluations, and even budgets. And they integrate health literacy into quality-improvement initiatives, patient safety initiatives, and provider competencies.

ATTRIBUTE 2: Health literate health care organizations develop a culture of active inquiry, partner in innovation, and invest in evaluations of operations improvements. Because the science of health literacy is not yet fully developed, health literate organizations need to partner with health literacy researchers from a number of fields to develop and implement interventions, to pilot successful interventions in real-world

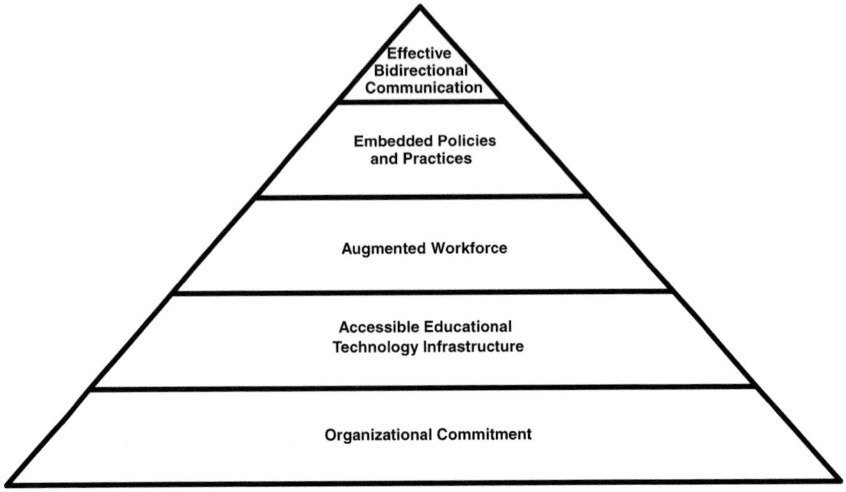

FIGURE 2-1 Framework for attributes for health literate health care organizations.
SOURCE: Schillinger and Keller, 2011.

settings, and to evaluate health literacy strategies and programming in real time, applying change as needed.

ATTRIBUTE 3: Health literate health care organizations measure and assess the health literacy environment and communication climate. They perform institutional assessments focused on the health literacy environment and the variety of communication and support systems in place. At both patient and organization levels, health literate health care organizations identify, track, and monitor health literacy metrics relevant to their organization. These organizations also track provider implementation of best practices in communication.

ATTRIBUTE 4: Health literate health care organizations commission and actively engage a health literacy advisory group that represents their target populations. A health literacy advisory group can have many functions, including

1. development and implementation of health literacy programming and strategies;
2. formulation of organizational policies around health literacy;
3. institutional health literacy reviews and environmental assessments; and
4. development and piloting of health information technology solutions, educational initiatives, and curricular materials.

BOX 2-2[a]
Proposed Attributes of a Health Literate Health Care Organization

1. Promote health literacy as an organizational responsibility.
2. Develop a culture of active inquiry, partner in innovation, and invest in rigorous evaluations of operations improvements.
3. Measure and assess the health literacy environment and communication climate.
4. Commission and actively engage a health literacy advisory group that represents the target populations.
5. Provide the infrastructure to avail frontline providers, patients, and families with a package of appropriate, high-quality educational supports and resources.
6. Leverage accessible health information technology (IT) to embed health literacy practices and support providers and patients.
7. Provide patient training and assistance around personal health records and health IT tools.
8. Foster an augmented and prepared workforce to promote health literacy.
9. Distribute resources to better meet the needs of the populations served.
10. Employ a higher standard to ensure understanding of high-risk decisions and high-risk transitions.
11. Prioritize medication safety and medication communication.
12. Make health plan and health insurance products more transparent and comprehensible.
13. Make systems more navigable and support patients and families in navigating the health care system.
14. Recognize social needs as medical concerns and connect people to community resources.
15. Create a climate in which question asking is encouraged and expected.
16. Develop and implement curricula to develop mastery of a threshold-level set of knowledge and skills.
17. Continually assess and track patient comprehension, skills, and ability to problem-solve around health conditions.
18. Recognize and accommodate additional barriers to communication.

---

[a] Following the workshop, members of the Workgroup on Attributes of a Health Literate Organization of the Roundtable on Health Literacy, using feedback provided on the paper, collapsed the number of attributes to 10 and published a discussion paper that articulates a rationale for these attributes and identifies the organizations that should use them. There is also a list of resources for organizations interested in taking action. The paper can be found at www.iom.edu/healthlit10attributes.

SOURCE: Schillinger and Keller, 2011.

ATTRIBUTE 5: Health literate health care organizations provide the infrastructure to avail frontline providers, patients, and families with a package of appropriate, high-quality educational supports and resources. Promoting patient comprehension and building skills requires high-quality human, technical, and pedagogical resources that are easily accessible across the organization. In addition to effective interpersonal communication, there is also a need to provide clearly written health information at the right time and place that embodies best practices in written information and applies health literacy principles. Health literate health care organizations ensure that there are multiple opportunities to interface with the health care team, to reinforce health education and self-management goals, and to assist with pre-visit planning and decision support.

The video decision aids developed by Volandes and colleagues for advanced care planning for Alzheimer disease[2] are good examples of best practice materials, Schillinger said. Another example can be found in the work of Project RED (Re-Engineered Discharge) at the Boston City Hospital,[3] which developed interactive, computer-based teaching tools based on health literacy principles. Health literate health care organizations have an instrumental role in influencing the marketplace of patient communication products by demanding rigorous testing with and adaptation for populations with limited health literacy, and in supporting the development of national certification standards for print and digital material that is accessible to these populations.

ATTRIBUTE 6: Health literate health care organizations leverage accessible health information technology (IT) to embed health literacy practices and support providers and patients. The health IT revolution has great potential to either narrow or widen the health literacy divide. An important role for health literate organizations, Schillinger said, will be to influence the marketplace of patient communication products, first by demanding that patient communication products be rigorously tested with and adapted for populations with limited health literacy and, second, by supporting the development of certification standards for print and digital material that is accessible to these populations.

---

[2] For a description see *Alzheimer Video Affects Care Preferences* in Clinical Psychiatry News. http://www.clinicalpsychiatrynews.com/search/search-single-view/alzheimer-s-video-affects-care-preferences/4c4fa54a41.html (accessed December 10, 2011).

[3] A description of Project RED can be found at http://www.bu.edu/fammed/projectred/ (accessed December 10, 2011).

ATTRIBUTE 7: Health literate health care organizations provide patient training and assistance around personal health records and health IT tools. There are many potential benefits of personal electronic health records (PEHRs). Patients can store and access personal health information, which provides them with additional points of interaction with providers. However, there remain multiple challenges in using PEHRs for populations with limited health literacy. A growing body of research shows that limited-literacy populations use personal electronic health records much less than their counterparts with adequate health literacy. This may partly be a question of access, but individuals with limited health literacy skills often also have low e-health literacy skills which prevent them from benefiting from such initiatives. Health literate organizations

1. involve populations with limited health literacy in the development and selection of electronic health record systems,
2. develop educational initiatives to orient and motivate patients in electronic health record use, and
3. ensure that information and education available on the personal health record can be accessed through interpersonal or alternative means for those who do not access the PEHR.

ATTRIBUTE 8: Health literate health care organizations foster an augmented and prepared workforce to promote health literacy. They develop a diversified workforce with expanded job descriptions for non-physician members which include a variety of educational roles—health educators, health coaches, navigators, medical assistants, peer educators, and expert educators. These are people who deeply understand health education, who help teach others how to teach, and who can tackle a challenging patient who does not appear to be acquiring the skills needed at the pace required to manage his or her condition. In order to ensure that all members of the health care team are prepared to employ best practices in communication during all patient interactions, organizations need to

1. prioritize recruiting health care team members who reflect the socio-demographic and linguistic profiles of the patient populations served;
2. provide health literacy and health communication training for all members of the integrated health team; and
3. provide more sophisticated training for the expert educators.

ATTRIBUTE 9: Health literate health care organizations distribute resources to better meet the needs of the populations served. The inverse care hypothesis, sometimes known as the inverse care law, was first described in the United Kingdom and states that the availability and quality of health care varies inversely with the needs of the population. Or, put more simply: "The more you need, the less you get." Health literate health care organizations understand that the inverse care law is especially relevant in the market-driven health care context. Therefore they allocate additional educational and communication resources to populations or to sites that have worse individual or population health outcomes that are attributable to limited health literacy. Furthermore, at the patient level such organizations provide intense and interactive communication proportional to the needs of its patients.

ATTRIBUTE 10: Health literate health care organizations employ a higher standard to ensure understanding of high-risk decisions and high-risk transitions. This involves identifying common high-risk decisions that require greater scrutiny, using standardized and well designed teaching tools for these decisions, and establishing health literacy practices (e.g., the teach-back method[4]) as part of the education and consent process. High-risk areas include consent for surgery; administration of medications with serious complications or "black box" warnings; and transitions in care, such as discharge from the hospital.

ATTRIBUTE 11: Health literate health care organizations prioritize medication safety and medication communication. They recognize that patients with limited health literacy have great difficulty with medication management and are more likely to misunderstand prescription labels and warning labels (Davis et al., 2006; Wolf et al., 2007) and more likely to make mistakes taking their medications (Lindquist et al., 2011; Sarkar et al., 2010). Systems and interventions are needed to advance medication safety and self management by, for example, efficiently incorporating medication reconciliation into the workflow, establishing guidelines and standards for uniform prescribing practices, and encouraging the use of plain language on the prescription label.

ATTRIBUTE 12: Health literate health care organizations make health plan and health insurance products more transparent and comprehensible. The enactment of the ACA will, Schillinger said, improve access to care through insurance reform, Medicaid expansion, and health insurance exchanges. To assist populations with limited health literacy fully realize the benefits of health care reform, it will be important to establish

[4] The teach-back method is a way of confirming patient understanding of what he or she needs to know and do by asking the patient to "teach back" the directions. http://www.ahrq.gov/qual/literacy/healthliteracytoolkit.pdf (accessed December 11, 2011).

methods to ensure that patients and families can access in-person support, that information about health benefit packages is understandable, and that better decision support is provided through such mechanisms as a plain-language summary of benefits, glossaries of terms, and culturally appropriate guides.

ATTRIBUTE 13: Health literate health care organizations make systems more navigable and support patients and families in navigating the health care system. They establish welcoming, shame-free environments where asking questions is encouraged. They offer assistance with literacy- and numeracy-related tasks. They implement system designs that can make the health system more navigable, such as the use of electronic referrals where the referring provider completes a detailed, electronic referral to the specialist that outlines all the information needed; in this way the patient is not responsible for providing all information. As part of making the system more navigable, health literate organizations perform environmental assessments to identify literacy barriers, signage problems, inconsistent labeling, or lack of available personnel for assistance.

ATTRIBUTE 14: Health literate health care organizations recognize social needs as medical concerns and connect people to community resources. They might partner with community resources, develop a clearinghouse of local resources, appoint a team member to be the expert in local resources, or partner with case managers and social workers to embed social services into health care delivery.

ATTRIBUTE 15: Health literate health care organizations create a climate in which question asking is encouraged and expected. They activate patients by implementing question-asking campaigns (e.g., the Ask Me 3 campaign[5] or Questions Are the Answers[6]) and encouraging allied staff to reinforce the asking of questions.

ATTRIBUTE 16: Health literate health care organizations develop and implement curricula to develop mastery of a threshold-level set of knowledge and skills. They use the following six principles in the development of these curricula (Baker et al., 2011):

---

[5] The Ask Me 3 campaign of the National Patient Safety Foundation encourages patients to ask such questions as, What is my main problem? What do I need to do? Why is it important for me to do this?

[6] Questions Are the Answers is a program developed by the Agency for Healthcare Research and Quality. More information can be found at http://www.ahrq.gov/questions/ (accessed December 11, 2011).

1. Define a limited set of critical learning goals and eliminate all other information that does not directly support the learning goals.
2. Present information in discrete, predetermined chunks.
3. Determine the optimal order for teaching the topics.
4. Develop plain language text to explain essential concepts for each goal and employ appropriate graphics to increase comprehension and recall.
5. Confirm understanding after each unit, perform tailored instruction until mastery is attained, and review previously learned concepts until stable mastery is achieved.
6. Link all instruction to a specific attitude, skill, or behavioral goal.

ATTRIBUTE 17: Health literate health care organizations continually assess and track patient comprehension, skills, and ability to problem-solve around health conditions. They assess and document patient comprehension and basic problem-solving abilities for health conditions that require self-management (e.g., congestive heart failure, diabetes, asthma, or anticoagulation). They put in place systems to connect individuals who have been identified as having continued educational needs with additional educational supports.

ATTRIBUTE 18: Health literate health care organizations recognize and accommodate additional barriers to communication. Patients with limited health literacy often face additional communication challenges. Most common among these are limited English proficiency and cognitive decline. There is compelling research that indicates that as many as one-third of the comprehension difficulties attributable to health literacy may actually be a consequence of subtle and undiagnosed cognitive problems, particularly among the elderly.

Hearing and visual impairment is common, particularly among low-income populations. A provider may think that a patient has limited health literacy when in reality he or she has bilateral wax impaction or a need for glasses. It is also possible that patients with limited health literacy have learning disabilities or learning differences that create specific problems with learning, problems that a teach-back method may not overcome. Or these patients may be burdened with mental health problems that prevented them from completing and succeeding in school. They may also have higher rates of depression that further impair recall and comprehension.

Health literate health care organizations develop many strategies to address additional communication barriers. They establish systems to identify and address communication disabilities. They provide extra support and case management to individuals with cognitive decline, and, if possible, they identify surrogates and family members to provide assistance. They uphold and implement cultural and linguistic standards, guidelines, and recommendations, recognizing the tremendous overlap between the importance of linguistic concordance and health literacy practice. And they recruit and cultivate a culturally and linguistically diverse staff.

Conclusion

This discussion, Schillinger said, has been a necessarily brief summary of the 21-page, single-spaced, highly referenced commissioned paper (see Appendix A) and, as such, provides only a superficial overview. The paper offers a set of attributes and foci for institutional investment by organizations striving to become more health literate. Many of the attributes apply to direct-service health organizations, but they can also be relevant to the broad range of institutions that now contribute to the health care system. The list, while long, is by no means exhaustive and should be viewed as either the beginning or the continuation of a conversation regarding how health care organizations can address health literacy at the institutional level. These attributes provide a view of how organizations should evolve to be more responsive to the needs of populations with limited health literacy in tangible ways.

DISCUSSION

Framework

Roundtable member Cindy Brach complimented Schillinger on the paper and asked whether one might collapse the 18 attributes to a smaller number and, if so, what the right number would be. Some of the attributes seem full of many kinds of things an organization can do, while others are more focused on a specific topic.

Schillinger replied that he and his coauthor struggled with deciding on the appropriate number. That is why the pyramid was created, he said—to begin to develop a framework. Attributes were then derived for each level of the framework: for organizational commitment, which is the foundation level of the pyramid; for the educational level, which is a very rich level and one in which health information technology can fit nicely; for the workforce level, which includes ways in which the workforce is trained and incentivized; for the embedded policies and practices level, which includes such things as embedding techniques for addressing high-risk situations in ways in which providers routinely interact with patients, whether it is clinically or online; and, finally, for the top level of the pyramid, bidirectional communication, which can be considered an outcome.

Roundtable chair George Isham said the framework that Schillinger presented, which begins with the organizational perspective of what it takes to succeed as an organization, has similarities to the Kaplan and Norton balanced scorecard approach[7] in which organizations consider four perspectives: financial, customer, business processes, and learning and growth. The idea is that the organization must be financially viable, relentlessly focused on the needs of the customer, with internal business processes that serve the organization's needs, and with a culture that continually learns from its experience and its contact with customers.

HealthPartners takes this approach and for health care translates the four perspectives into people, health, experience, and affordability. If one relentlessly focuses on improving the health and experiences of the people one serves, Isham said, one is inevitably led to think about health disparities and health literacy. Another framework that resonates with the attributes presented at the workshop is the one presented in the IOM report *Crossing the Quality Chasm* (2001). That report lists six aims for care provided by health care organizations: Care should be safe, timely, effective, efficient, equitable, and patient-centered. In the 10 years since that report was published, there has been insufficient progress on making care equitable or patient-centered, Isham said, but nonetheless the report is extremely valuable in helping one think about how to move forward in these areas.

The attributes paper presented at the workshop also helps one think critically and thoughtfully about the relationship of health literacy and health disparities, Isham said, and such thinking can contribute to obtaining equitable and patient-centered care. The paper also provides ideas about how one might make progress in reducing disparities by addressing issues of poor health literacy.

Roundtable member Paul Schyve said that one needs to think about the pyramid and attributes as conceptual: What story do they tell that will stimulate changes in the health care system and in policymakers understanding? The story is that the system is far behind on achieving the six aims of quality care, particularly the ones dealing with equity and patient-centeredness. How do the attributes relate to improvements in these areas?

Roundtable member Benard Dreyer agreed that the paper is a critical contribution to thinking about health literacy and quality improvement.

---

[7] The balanced scorecard approach "is a strategic approach and performance management system that enables organizer's to translate a company's vision and strategy into implementation, working from 4 perspectives": financial, customer, business process, and learning and growth. http://www.valuebasedmanagement.net/methods_balancedscorecard.html (accessed December 13, 2011).

As the pyramid shows, organizational commitment is the basis for a health literate organization. The lack of that commitment is the reason so little progress has been made, he said. Dreyer's concern is that organizations will decide to pick one or two attributes rather than trying to do something with each. Is the pyramid a stepladder? he asked Schillinger. Does an organization have to go from one to the next? Are there critical things that need to be done at one level before going to the next step?

Schillinger said that there is overlap among the levels of the pyramid. Furthermore, it is not feasible to attempt to address all 18 attributes simultaneously. As for where one should focus first, he said it is likely that finances will drive many of the decisions about how to proceed with the attributes. An organization may try to first address those attributes that it believes will have the greatest return on investment. If one takes the risk-management perspective, then high-risk decision moments may be the place to start. High-risk decision moments are also very palpable places to intervene at the level of the provider and would demonstrate that the organization has committed to doing things differently. Or the organization might decide to focus on high-risk conditions such as congestive heart failure or on transitions in care.

The key question is from what perspective the organization will approach the attributes: a clinical, financial, population health, or public health perspective? From the public health perspective, for example, one would want to embed practices and use a universal-precautions approach in order to have incremental improvements applicable to the greatest number of patients and, thereby, improve population health. What an organization chooses to do will depend on decision making at the executive level in terms of what that organization wants to achieve.

General Comments

Roundtable member Leonard Epstein said that the paper neatly puts together in one place what needs to be accomplished at an organizational level in order to achieve effective health care communication. It would also be helpful, he said, to articulate the major components of effective health communication. Health literacy is obviously one component, as are effective cross cultural communication, use of trained interpreters and translators, and use of plain language. These need to be emphasized more, Epstein said.

Roundtable member Winston Wong said that the attributes presented resonated with what Kaiser has been exploring, particularly in terms of using the electronic health record to capture utilization information and track demographic profiles of users. Another aspect of the attributes that Kaiser has been examining relates to health equity or health disparities.

The organization is looking at specific ways it can intervene in situations with measurable clinical disparities and is incorporating aspects of health literacy into the strategies for approaching different population groups. Finally, he said that the attribute concerning assessing and tracking patient comprehension for conditions requiring self-management captures some of the work Kaiser is doing with different chronic disease management strategies.

Roundtable member Yolanda Partida said that the paper seemed to address health care organizations only and asked where the public health or community level fits. What about health organizations that do community-based work?

Schillinger replied that there is no question that public health has a critical role to play, particularly in integrated systems that are public delivery systems such as the New York Health and Hospitals Corporation. There are a range of issues that need to be addressed around public health communication and public health in clinical connectivity. However, the charge from the roundtable for preparing this paper specified that the focus was to be health care organizations, not public health entities.

Roundtable member Scott Ratzan asked Schillinger to think about the idea of integrating a checklist into Attribute 17 ("Continually assess and track patient comprehension, skills, and ability to problem-solve around health conditions."). A simple checklist for congestive heart failure, diabetes, asthma and other chronic diseases could be used to assess whether patients are, for example, practicing the most important behaviors for their conditions. The safe surgery checklist developed by the World Health Organization[8] is an example of such a checklist. Or, he asked, are the chronic conditions too complex for such an approach?

Schillinger said that he believes developing such checklists would indeed be complicated and would require significant work to define the crucial pieces that need to be included, but that such checklists would be a major contribution.

Linda Harris, another roundtable member, suggested that in thinking about attributes of a health literate organization it might be useful to use such language and concepts as productive interactions in the Chronic Care Model,[9] patient-centered care, the medical home, and accountable

[8] The checklist can be viewed at http://www.who.int/patientsafety/safesurgery/en/ (accessed December 13, 2011).

[9] The model can be found at http://www.improvingchroniccare.org/index.php?p=the_chronic_care_model&s=2 (accessed December 13, 2011).

care organizations (ACOs).[10] Organizations and individuals may not relate to the term "health literate organization," but they do relate to the other terms. It would be useful to create a conceptual map that shows how these concepts correlate with the attributes.

Roundtable member Ruth Parker said there is an opportunity to frame the discussion more broadly in order to help those who provide health care see that a health literate organization is one that values health and values sharing that with populations and individuals. This means not wasting money and resources as well as being accountable. Accountable care organizations were mentioned earlier, but no one yet understands what that means. We have an opportunity to advance the national conversation about ACOs; that is, a necessary element of an ACO is to be a health literate organization. There is nothing more patient-centered than health literacy, Parker said.

Roundtable member Sharon Barrett said that the paper provides a comprehensive view of what the attributes of a health literate organization look like. What is the next step? Can one pull out from these the "how to"? This will be important, she said, because a number of organizations are going to begin to look at what they can do to become health literate organizations. Perhaps there is some way to look at this as a continuum, since it is unlikely that an organization can accomplish everything mentioned in the paper.

Schillinger said that the paper authors explicitly tried not to create the perception that each of the attributes has to be accomplished immediately. The paper is focused on goals and recognizes that a great deal of work needs to be done between where things stand now and where things will stand in the future. Becoming a health literate organization is a process and achieving each attribute moves the organization along the continuum closer to becoming a health literate organization.

Isham concluded by saying that the tangible suggestions offered in the paper provide a clear way to think about how to align incentives for organizations so that they do the right thing and succeed as an organization.

---

[10] "An ACO is a network of doctors and hospitals that shares responsibility for providing care to patients. In the new law, an ACO would agree to manage all of the health care needs of a minimum of 5,000 Medicare beneficiaries for at least three years." http://www.kaiserhealthnews.org/stories/2011/january/13/aco-accountable-care-organization-faq.aspx (accessed December 13, 2011).

REFERENCES

Baker, D. W., D. A. Dewalt, D. Schillinger, V. Hawk, B. Ruo, K. Bibbins-Domingo, M. Weinberger, A. Macabasco-O'Connell, and M. Pignone. 2011. "Teach to goal": Theory and design principles of an intervention to improve heart failure self-management skills of patients with low health literacy. *Journal of Health Communication* 16(Suppl 3):73–88.

Davis, T. C., M. S. Wolf, P. F. Bass, 3rd, M. Middlebrooks, E. Kennen, D. W. Baker, C. L. Bennett, R. Durazo-Arvizu, A. Bocchini, S. Savory, and R. M. Parker. 2006. Low literacy impairs comprehension of prescription drug warning labels. *Journal of General Internal Medicine* 21(8):847–851.

IOM (Institute of Medicine). 2001. *Crossing the Quality Chasm: A New Health System for the 21st Century.* Washington, DC: National Academy Press.

Lindquist, L. A., L. Go, J. Fleisher, N. Jain, E. Friesema, and D. W. Baker. 2011. Relationship of health literacy to intentional and unintentional non-adherence of hospital discharge medications. *Journal of General Internal Medicine* 27(2):173–178.

Sarkar, U., A. J. Karter, J. Y. Liu, N. E. Adler, R. Nguyen, A. Lopez, and D. Schillinger. 2010. The literacy divide: Health literacy and the use of an Internet-based patient portal in an integrated health system—results from the Diabetes Study of Northern California (DISTANCE). *Journal of Health Communications* 15(Suppl 2):183–196.

Schillinger, D., and D. Keller. 2011. *The Other Side of the Coin: Attributes of a Health Literate Health Care Organization*. PowerPoint presentation at the Institute of Medicine Workshop on Attributes of a Health Literate Organization. Washington, DC. November 16.

Wolf, M. S., T. C. Davis, W. Shrank, D. N. Rapp, P. F. Bass, U. M. Connor, M. Clayman, and R. M. Parker. 2007. To err is human: Patient misinterpretations of prescription drug label instructions. *Patient Education and Counseling* 67(3):293–300.

3

Reaction Panel 1

PUBLIC HOSPITAL SYSTEM

Lauren W. Johnston, RN, M.P.A., NEA-BC, FACHE
New York City Health and Hospital Corporation

The mission of the New York City Health and Hospital Corporation (HHC) is to provide comprehensive health services regardless of a patient's ability to pay. In fulfilling its mission, Johnston said, HHC seeks to promote the fullest meaning of health: total physical, mental, and social well-being. HHC is the largest municipal organization in the country, she said. It has revenues of about $7 billion, and it includes 11 acute-care facilities, 4 long-term care facilities, 6 diagnostic and treatment centers, 80 other community health clinics, and a home care agency. HHC also has its own managed care health plan and 40,000 employees. It uses an employed physician model.

Annually, HHC has about 1 million emergency department visits, 5 million clinic visits, and 25,000 babies delivered. About 70 percent of the behavioral health population being cared for in New York City is cared for at HHC. The population it serves is ethnically and culturally diverse, with many patients being recently arrived immigrants. During 2010 HHC had 450,000 uninsured visits, and approximately 40 percent of those seen were undocumented immigrants. Translation services are routinely provided in more than 100 languages.

No two hospitals or facilities have the same distribution of languages or culture. Many HHC hospitals have been the cornerstones of their communities for more than a century, and many of them are the largest employers in their areas. HHC provides a safety net not only for health care, but many times also for financial counseling, legal issues, and family support. This is important because if a patient does not know where he is going to sleep that night or isn't sure whether he will eat, he is not listening to instructions about such things as weighing himself every day.

Health literacy includes more than just health information and health services, Johnston said. It is about helping people live their lives. For example, about two years ago the contractor handling the HHC health information system experienced a breach in the security of information for about 150,000 people. That contractor offered the 150,000 patients a toll-free number to call for information and free credit reports for a year. But the offer was all in English. Of course, the patients immediately came to HHC staff with the letter—an entire page all written in legalese and barely understandable to English speakers—and said, What are we supposed to do with this?

HHC set up a system to help the patients. Staff members explained what the letter meant and provided telephone support because the contractor was unaware of the patients' language needs and only offered telephone support in English. Then, when the credit reports were delivered, the patients brought them in to HHC to find out what those reports meant. That is an example of health care literacy, Johnston said.

HHC has attempted to address many of the attributes described in the commissioned paper. Although not fully successful, the organization is on the path described. HHC sees the following attributes as top priorities:

- Establish promoting health literacy as an organizational responsibility.
- Foster an augmented and prepared workforce to promote health literacy.
- Distribute resources to better meet the needs of the populations served.

Several initiatives are important as the base from which HHC will help provide the support patients need to become health literate, including initiatives aimed at transparency and patient-centeredness. One of HHC's cornerstones is transparency, Johnston said. In 2007 HHC president Alan Aviles wrote an article explaining why HHC publishes patient outcomes and patient satisfaction results on its website—it is part of becoming a transparent organization, to which HHC is fully committed. Furthermore, all of the ambulatory care sites are approved by the National Committee for Quality Assurance at Level 3, the highest level of approval, as patient-centered medical homes, delivering high-quality primary care.

In terms of the attribute "leverage accessible health information technology (IT) to embed health literacy practices and support providers and patients," HHC meets the information technology meaningful-use requirements, which include education of patients. Medication and patient medication communication have been made a priority (Attribute 11), and there are well-established offices for culturally and linguistically appropriate services (CLAS) with translation services at all points of care.

HHC is also moving forward with workforce development and is currently undertaking an assessment concerning workforce development. It is probable that there are not enough educators. A number of staff members could provide education, but they are currently prevented from doing so because of the press of daily tasks. The aim of the assessment is to be sure that staff members are being used most effectively. It will be important to include all staff in this effort—physicians, nurses, other health care disciplines, volunteers, and peer coaches.

There are many challenges that HHC faces in its efforts to improve the literacy of its patients and staff. In the area of information technology, for example, many vendors can offer programs only in English and Spanish, so those programs have to be supplemented. While the organization has an office of CLAS and translation services at every facility, this does not mean that staff members are aware of all important cultural perspectives. But one must be able to talk with patients before one can understand their cultures. Efforts are also being made to raise everyone's expectations about the ability of staff members to communicate with patients. Unfortunately, the organization was faced with a $1 billion deficit which definitely affects what can be achieved in educating the workforce and providing the time needed to increase effective communication with patients. Other challenges include the transitory nature of the patient population—as individuals improve their financial status, they move to other places—as well as the need to overcome the inherent lack of trust among many patients in anyone functioning in an official capacity.

While there may be incentives for moving forward with programs and policies to become a more health literate organization, the main difficulty is really one of complexity, Johnston said. What should be the priorities? How does one choose what to work on first? What do we know about what will work and what will not work? Just because a program works in one community or one hospital doesn't mean it will work the same in another. How do we know what to change? Return on investment is an important criterion in making decisions about what to do.

There is not anything in the commissioned paper that is undesirable, Johnston said, although there is a great deal that will be a challenge to implement at this time. "Develop a culture of active inquiry, partner in innovation, invest in rigorous evaluations of operations improvements" is a difficult attribute to implement, she said. The immediate focus is to get everyone to do what is needed at the time it is needed. Another attribute, "Provide patient training and assistance around personal health records and health IT tools," is a stretch for the population served by the organization since people do not always have reliable access to technology. And other than during patient visits, it is extremely difficult to "continually assess and track patient comprehension, skills, and ability to problem-solve around health conditions," another worthwhile but difficult attribute. With the patient-centered medical home,[1] the intention is to add to patients' choices on how the organization communicates with them. Rather than just relying on face-to-face communication with physicians, for example, if a patient says the best way to communicate is by cell phone, that is how communication will be conducted.

There is enormous need to improve health literacy. From HHC's point of view the attributes would benefit from specificity, prioritization, and identification of costs. This would help organizations develop plans for implementing programs to achieve these attributes. Of course, Johnston concluded, there will always be the question of how much can be done, given the resources available and the benefit expected. Changing the organization and workforce culture requires major effort, but it is effort that HHC is committed to giving.

PUBLIC CLINIC

Debra Dever, RN, BSN, MN
Loudon Community Health Center

Loudon Community Health Center in Leesburg, Virginia is a federally qualified health center (FQHC).[2] The FQHC model has existed for 45 years in the United States. It is a model designed to provide access to health care services for low-income, uninsured, and underinsured people. The program began in inner-city urban areas and in extremely rural areas

[1] "A Patient-Centered Medical Home is a team-based model of care led by a personal physician who provides continuous and coordinated care throughout a patient's lifetime to maximize health outcomes." http://www.medscape.com/viewarticle/589670 (accessesd April 1, 2012).

[2] "Federally qualified health centers (FQHCs) include all organizations receiving grants under Section 330 of the Public Health Service Act, certain tribal organizations, and FQHC Look-Alikes. FQHCs qualify for enhanced reimbursement from Medicare and Medicaid, as well as other benefits." Five requirements of an FHQC are that they serve an underserved area or population; offer a sliding fee scale; provide comprehensive services; have an ongoing quality assurance program; and have a governing board of directors. http://www.raconline.org/topics/clinics/fqhc.php (accessed December 15, 2011).

where there was no access to health care services. Today there are more than 1,000 FQHCs across the United States (Kaiser Family Foundation, 2011).

Loudon County is the richest county in the nation, Dever said. A large influx of immigrants over the past 10 years has contributed to the 800 percent growth in population. It is currently estimated that there are 40,000 uninsured residents in Loudon County, many of whom are undocumented immigrants.

Loudon Community Health Center is four years old. It began with a staff of five and one physician. The center has served 10,000 patients and has 7,000 active patients at two sites. The population served by the center is very poor. Ninety percent of those served are at 200 percent or less of the federal poverty level (FPL); of those, about 60 percent are under 100 percent of the FPL. Those served come from over 80 different countries; 55 percent are Hispanic, and 45 percent of patients require an interpreter or other language assistance. The most common diagnosis among the adult population is diabetes, followed by hypertension, then hyperlipidemia, with depression as the fourth most common diagnosis.

The center provides primary medical care and preventive care. It has family practice, board certified providers, and some mid-level providers. There is a psychiatrist on staff and two mental health counselors to provide mandated mental health services. The mandated dental care is provided through a referral system, and access to radiology services is accomplished through agreements with off-site providers. There is a professor of pharmacy from a school of pharmacy who is on site half time, and the school's senior pharmacy students rotate through the center. There is a medications program to provide access to needed medications and an in-house laboratory.

The mission of the center is to provide all of the residents of the community, especially those who are uninsured and medically underserved, with access to comprehensive, cost-effective, high-quality, culturally competent primary and preventive health care. The center is committed to being culturally competent. Its vision is to be a model primary health care organization, to eliminate health disparities in the community, and to become the medical home of choice in Loudon County. To accomplish its mission and vision the center provides whatever enabling services are needed to overcome barriers to obtaining services. In Loudon County the number-one barrier is a lack of transportation, and the second is the language barrier.

Which attributes are more relevant to the center? Of major importance is the attribute "Provide the infrastructure to avail frontline providers, patients, and families with a package of appropriate, high-quality educational supports and resources." This is a major challenge. The center has educational materials in English and Spanish; the challenge is instead with other languages. To prepare materials in other languages takes time, and that is one thing that is a major barrier for center staff: There just isn't enough time.

Another important attribute is "Leverage accessible health information technology (IT) to embed health literacy practices and support providers and patients." The center is working very hard to effectively use its electronic health record, but the demands of time and resources and the need to standardize across the Virginia health centers made it impossible to involve the community in the development of the system. The center is investigating the establishment of a portal to overcome some of the difficulties, and to that end staff members wrote a grant to obtain resources to hire an informatics person. Because it will be very difficult to identify all the data needed to become a certified medical home, informatics expertise will be critical.

One top priority is medication safety and medication communication. The center currently asks all patients to bring their medications with them to their appointments. Given the center's relationship with the school of pharmacy, a knowledgeable person is generally available to meet with the patients to explain their medications or to act as consultants to the center's other providers. The center is also eligible for what is called a 340B pharmacy.[3]

The challenge is the diversity of the population served. How does one ensure that individuals from all the different cultures that make up the center's patient population really understand how to take their medications appropriately or recognize that it is important to do so? Furthermore, some patients who have just entered the United States have been taking herbs or other unknown medications. It can take more than one visit and several hours to decipher what they have been taking and try to develop plans for their future medication use. Another challenge is creating a climate in which asking questions is encouraged and expected. The teach-back method and Ask Me Three are very intriguing approaches that will be helpful as the center educates its providers and nursing staff.

The center is absolutely committed to undertaking activities to become a health literate organization. The challenge in implementing

---

[3] "Section 340B of the Public Health Service Act (created under Section 602 of the Veterans Health Care Act of 1992), which requires pharmaceutical manufacturers participating in the Medicaid program to enter into a second agreement with the Secretary under which the manufacturer agrees to provide discounts on covered outpatient drugs purchased by specified government-supported facilities, called 'covered entities,' that serve the nation's most vulnerable patient populations." http://www.cjaonline.net/events/SustSeries/Calls/Call20080918/OverviewSection340B2.pdf (accessed December 16, 2011).

these attributes is that the center has significant productivity expectations that have to be met. The question then becomes how, even with support staff, can what needs to be done be accomplished in a 15-minute visit. Other challenges include resources, manpower, expertise, and money. The federal budget for community health centers was cut earlier this year by $330 million. That meant a $215,000 cut for the center.

In terms of incentives to implement activities, the major one is financial resources, but another thing that would help would be to be able to learn about the types of programs and services that have worked in other facilities. It would be helpful if there were standardized education materials and checklists available so that each facility would not be reinventing everything.

None of the attributes listed in the paper are undesirable. Some of them are more difficult than others, such as developing metrics, particularly in the center setting. And there is no way the center would have the resources to employ a health literacy officer.

Dever concluded by saying that the attributes are in line with the center's mission and vision and that the commitment is there to implement programs and activities to achieve these attributes. What it comes down to, she said, is possessing adequate resources.

DISCUSSION

Roundtable member Patrick McGarry noted that both speakers highlighted the attribute related to a workforce prepared to promote health literacy. How is such a workforce developed? Are there job descriptions that have health literacy included? Are there criteria used to assess whether a workforce is health literate? Are continuing medical education (CME) credits or continuing education units (CEUs) required?

Johnston responded that HHC is still in the assessment stage. The organization is trying to support the workforce. It does not require CME credits but is working to assure that CME programs are available. It is important to emphasize that the need for a health literate workforce is not confined to physicians. Health literacy is important for everyone. HHC also provides CEUs for nurses and has the ability to include other professions in continuing education. But, again, the organization is still at the point of determining not only what staff is able to do, but also what they are actually doing. The assessment has found, for example, that just about everyone on staff answers the telephone or makes appointments. Yet some staff should be focusing elsewhere, such as on medication education and teach-back. The organization is in the process of revising the job descriptions so that they better reflect what members of each profession should be doing to work at the peak of their licensure. The problem is one of resources: The work has to be done yet there are not enough people to do it.

Dever said that at Loudon Community Health Center cultural competence and cultural sensitivity are built into the job descriptions at every level. When staff go through hiring interviews, questions are asked to ascertain how the interviewee might react in certain situations requiring a cultural perspective. There is also mandated cultural competency training for which the clinic is closed for a day so that staff members can attend the training session. Health literacy is the next area to be targeted. Finances are the limiting factor because it is financially difficult to close the clinic in order to conduct the training. There is online training available, and staff members are encouraged to participate in that.

Roundtable member Winston Wong complimented the organizations of both speakers for being dedicated to serving the needs of the underserved. It appears that both organizations think not only of the patients that enter the facilities but also about overall community needs. To what extent, he asked, does each of the organizations think about the health literacy needs of the community? Is there a way in which that can be systematically assessed? And how can those needs be addressed?

Johnson responded that HHC is grounded in its communities. Currently every facility has a community advisory board, and each of those tends to be politically active locally. However, sometimes that means that the information that reaches the organization has been screened. Therefore, in an effort to reach out to the communities themselves, many of the facilities have begun holding patient forums and including patients in root cause analysis[4] and on patient safety rounds. One of the facilities, for example, has begun work on community-oriented patients care, but it is a long process. The patients and the community must trust the facility. Many patients and community members are not ready to talk about the issues they think are important, so efforts at establishing partnerships with individuals and community organizations are under way. There are also efforts aimed at determining patient satisfaction.

Dever said that FQHCs are required to conduct a complete community-needs assessment every 5 years. While the Loudon center's assessment has not focused specifically on health literacy, it has looked at the diversity and the cultural needs of the community. Furthermore, the satisfaction surveys include questions about whether patients understood what their problem was, whether they received explanations they understood,

[4] A reoccurring problem makes it is important to determine the actual cause of the problem so that that cause can be removed, thereby preventing the situation from occurring again. This is called root cause analysis. http://www.systems-thinking.org/rca/rootca.htm. (accessed December 21, 2011).

and if they know their treatment plans. FQHCs are also required to have a board of directors of which at least 51 are percent community members. This means that the board is incredibly diverse, with low-income individuals from many different countries. They are, therefore, able to identify challenges in access and other barriers.

Schillinger noted that both Johnston and Dever had been talking about safety net systems—one of which is immense and the other smaller. Both have taken the universal approach to health literacy and other challenges, since nearly everyone in both facilities is facing those challenges. On the one hand, these attributes fit with the missions of each organization, thereby making it easier to build the attributes into the system because those attributes align with the mission. On the other hand, there is a great challenge because achieving the attributes requires reallocating resources, but the major challenge both organizations face is the amount of resources coming into the system. Other organizations, Schillinger continued, are not explicitly safety-net organizations and may have more leeway in discretionary decision making.

Isham said that the entire health care system is at a challenging point. The commissioned paper presents a set of recommendations that could be viewed as optional add-ons or as critical and important. Which view an organization takes, which choices it makes, is all the more important in terms of determining what the organization currently is doing versus what it could do to be more effective in meeting patients' needs.

REFERENCE

Kaiser Family Foundation. 2011. *Number of Federally Funded Federally Qualified Health Centers, 2010.* Available at http://www.statehealthfacts.org/comparemaptable.jsp?cat=8&ind=424 (accessed December 15, 2011).

4

Reaction Panel 2

PHYSICIAN PRIVATE PRACTICE

Isabel Hoverman, M.D.
Austin Internal Medicine Associates

Austin Internal Medicine Associates is a four-physician internal medicine practice. Its patient population, Hoverman said, is fairly heterogeneous—many are well educated, but there are also a number of disadvantaged patients, including a number of people with chronic psychiatric illness and mental retardation and a large number of Medicare patients. Most of the attributes described in the commissioned paper are doable, she said, although they are probably not doable in a small private practice, and more than 40 percent of physicians practice in small groups.

Organizational commitment is a very important attribute, she said, as are policies and procedures to support health literacy efforts. Health literacy is a team-based effort. For example, the first level of contact in her practice is the front desk. The practice has tried to simplify its registration forms so they can be understood at a very basic level, and patient information brochures have all been rewritten to remove as much jargon as possible.

Questions concerning what is covered in the many different health plans present particular challenges to the managers in the practice: What is the co-pay? Is the practice listed as a primary provider? Does the patient need a referral? Few patients know what their insurance covers or what their out-of-pocket expenses will be. Talking about a bill for services involves a whole separate language: co-pays, deductibles, usual and allowable fees, covered and non-covered services. This is language that few other than those who use it every day in their work understand.

Over the years the practice has struggled with employees who are frustrated by patients who did not understand their benefits or the terms of their health plans. "Making health care plans and insurance products more transparent and comprehensible"—one of the attributes mentioned in the paper—is a huge priority for the practice as it would save significant time and energy for both patients and the practice.

Another important attribute is "Foster an augmented and prepared workforce to promote health literacy." The health literacy of the staff can be a barrier to having a health literate practice. The practice started conducting interviews with staff members, asking simple questions. Discussions were held and then the staff was asked to write down what the message of the discussion was. One finding was that many of the staff could not triage a telephone call. Also, while many employees are sympathetic to patients' needs, they may not have an understanding of what patients are asking. Therefore, the policy of this practice is that no front-desk office staff member can take messages with clinical content. The front office staff asks what the call is regarding, so that if there is an emergency or if the patient is ill and needs more than an appointment, a nurse or a doctor handles it right away. The practice has also looked at the health literacy of its medical assistants. Because the term "medical" is in the name of their position, patients often assume that they are able to perform at a higher level, but these are really entry level jobs with minimal training. It is important to make sure the medical assistants have the knowledge to function appropriately.

Many patients are computer literate, but a large number do not feel comfortable with the Internet as a source of information or do not have easy access to the Internet. Many patients are unable to conduct reliable searches for disease information. Those who are slightly more computer literate tend to conduct a broad search and then have trouble separating information that is evidence-based from that which is not. The practice uses MedlinePlus.gov as well as specialty society websites and disease-specific sites run by related associations (e.g., the American Diabetes Association and the American Cancer Society) as information sources for patients. The practice could do a better job of providing patients with a broader list of useful Internet sites that provide reliable information.

While being able to access one's own health records via computer is attractive, it is difficult to imagine that this will occur widely in the near future, Hoverman said. Most electronic health records (EHRs) in the medical community are in a format to satisfy CPT coding guidelines and thus justify billing. Often important and useful information about why the patient was seen, what the recommendations for treatment were, or what the patients were told is either missing or hidden in pages of text that summarize previous treatments or in family and social history that is documented but does not change from visit to visit.

Addressing the issue of important attributes on which a small physician practice might place priority, Hoverman said that medication safety and medication communication are paramount. Communicating with patients using such approaches as the "Ask Me Three" campaign is both possible and desirable. The practice uses checklists to a certain extent but could do a better job. Medical personnel try to use simple language by, for example, talking about the importance of "checking one's sugar" rather than the importance of "glucose testing."

There are several major barriers medical practices face in implementing the attributes. The greatest barrier to addressing health literacy, for instance, is not recognizing that there is a problem. Another barrier is the limited time available to spend with patients. Some patients have low English proficiency or differing cultural or personal beliefs. Others have cognitive decline, hearing or visual impairment, or mental health problems. These barriers make effective communication more difficult and time consuming. Ultimately, the focus needs to be on providing patient-centered care, and that means meeting the health literacy needs of the patients served, Hoverman concluded.

PHARMACY PRACTICE

Darren Townzen, R.Ph., M.B.A.
Wal-Mart Stores, Inc.

Wal-Mart Stores Inc. operates about 4,500 pharmacies across the United States, Townzen said, and within the health and wellness division there are also clinics and vision centers. These clinics are not owned by Walmart, but rather they are leased to partners in the local health care system. Each pharmacy and each clinic is required to have an electronic medical record and to transmit prescriptions electronically.

Many of the attributes described in the commissioned paper did not seem to apply to a retail setting, Townzen said. However, four definitely did. These are

1. embedding health literacy practices into health information technology (IT) to support providers and patients;
2. providing patient training and assistance around personal health records and health IT tools;

3. prioritizing medications safety and medication communication; and
4. recognizing and making accommodations for additional barriers to communication.

Focusing on attributes related to health IT is a priority for Walmart because it allows use of new and existing technology to aid in the pharmacy mission. For example, one of the things Walmart pharmacies do is to text-message a customer when his or her prescription is ready. The company is also developing more meaningful messages, such as letting patients know when they are late on chronic medications—something that is good for the patient and provides a positive return on investment to the pharmacy.

The pharmacies gave customers the option of receiving either a text message or a telephone call. Most people wanted to receive a call, and the hypothesis is that people believed they would have to pay to receive the text message but would not for the call. Such a perception is a barrier to the use of technology.

Providing patient training and assistance around personal health records and health IT tools is another attribute that is important to Walmart. Patients can access their prescriptions through Walmart's website, but this technology is not being used. And Walmart employees rarely use their own personal health records, even though all were provided with them. Trying to motivate a customer, patient, or employee to use this technology is difficult, but such use, if it could become standard, could be extremely beneficial.

Another high-priority attribute is medication safety and medication communication. Pharmacists view this as a social responsibility, Townzen said. One approach to improving medication safety and communication would be to develop a more health literate prescription label. Another would be to work with physicians so that they do not view the pharmacist as a mere dispenser of medication but rather as an active partner in providing high-quality care to patients.

An adequately trained workforce is also key. Pharmacy staff members should reflect the community so that they can better communicate with those who use the pharmacy. Interpreters are needed to aid in increasing patient understanding and comprehension. Certainly the written information provided with prescriptions is unlikely to be read or used by patients. A much more strategic approach to providing information is needed.

Internally, Walmart is developing communication systems for patients with limited English proficiency and addressing how to counsel a patient. One challenge to becoming a health literate organization is competing priorities. Some projects are compliance-driven because of regulations.

Others are business-dictated projects. It will be of major importance to determine the best way to distribute available resources so as to make sure that pharmacies are delivering good value rather than just satisfying a rule or regulation, Townzen concluded.

DISCUSSION

Roundtable member Paul Schyve said he was stuck by Townzen's comment that implementation will depend on competing priorities and on expense. The roundtable is focused on how important health literacy is, but in practice settings people are faced with many important things that must be done, many of which are not currently being done. How do organizations, whether private-practice medical offices, Wal-Mart Stores, or a health plan and delivery system, make decisions about priorities and about where to put resources?

Townzen responded that the Walmart system is attempting to develop a more robust informatics strategy. Health benefits are achieved when patients stay in compliance with their therapy and they are getting their prescriptions filled on time.

Hoverman said that change in her practice required a change in culture at all levels. It is not a question of, Can we spend X dollars? Change must come from the leadership, which means that the leadership must understand the problem. But changing culture is very difficult. One advantage of having taken care of many of the patients for a very long time is that the staff members know the patients, their families, and their problems and are more sympathetic, which is a big plus in facilitating needed change.

Isham said that for his health plan, decisions must fit into a chain of logic and rationale that allows taking advantage of the resources that already exist for the purpose of meeting the identified needs. Choices need to facilitate superior patient experiences as well as having a value proposition for the health plans, both medical and dental. It is not a matter of whether one has more or less in these challenging times, but rather it is a matter of how to redeploy existing resources to meet these very important needs. What the commissioned paper does is point the way, very specifically and tangibly, to how one can make the arguments for redeployment.

Cynthia Baur from the U.S. Centers for Disease Control and Prevention asked what innovative strategies Wal-Mart Stores is pursuing to achieve the attributes of health literacy. Townzen responded that making the attributes a priority within the organization would motivate the creation of innovative strategies. This requires getting the right people to focus on the issue. The practice management system is designed around pulling people from the field—those on the front line—in order to come up with solutions.

Isham said his impression is that organizations like Walmart are focused on meeting the needs of the customers or patients at an affordable cost. There is tremendous potential for such organizations to address the issues of health literacy. Such organizations can challenge those in the more conventional health care system to be more creative.

Roundtable member Benard Dreyer asked whether the personal health records kept by Walmart contain the kinds of information that patients are likely to want to know or whether they are records of only a small portion of the patient's health. If the latter, perhaps that is why the records are not accessed. Another possible reason for lack of use might be the way in which the information is presented. Is it presented in a format that a patient can understand and use? Electronic medical records are being promulgated across the United States, but they may well be in a format or use language that is not understandable and usable by the patient. That seems to be what the attribute concerning electronic health records is trying to convey.

Townzen replied that the personal health record contains a record of all prescriptions filled within one of Walmart's facilities. It also contains all of the information needed for medical billing and processing. Users are also allowed to enter information themselves, including over-the-counter medications used and other information they think is important. And notifications are sent when something has been updated in the record. In terms of usability, it may be that the company to which the system has been outsourced needs to conduct some focus groups or other investigations into the record's usability.

Roundtable member Sharon Barrett asked if Townzen could describe more fully what Wal-Mart Stores is doing for its employees in terms of its health insurance packages. Is there some kind of training to help them become more health literate or knowledgeable about what an appropriate packages for them might be?

Townzen said that there is an internal website that is very easy to navigate that provides all kinds of information for employees. It is still a work in progress, but Walmart hopes it will become a very useful tool.

Roundtable member Cindy Brach asked both Townzen and Hoverman what their overall reactions were to the attributes presented in the commissioned paper. Did the paper make you reflect on your own organization and ask yourself how it is doing and whether it is a health literate organization? Did it inspire you to think about new ways in which you might stretch yourselves to take on something new, to address some attribute that you are not currently addressing? Did it provide you with any guidance on how you might do this? And, finally, do you have any suggestions on what might be missing from the paper or what should be changed?

Hoverman replied that, as she had stated in her presentation, she was inspired by the report. She had never heard about some of the tools mentioned, such as the Ask Me Three campaign, but she was excited about integrating into her practice. However, she said, there are two very different kinds of audiences for this paper—the audience composed of large organizations, such as the New York City Health and Hospital Corporation and Wal-Mart Stores, and the audience that is composed of small groups, such as the physician group practice or the independent pharmacy. Certainly there are some attributes that all of these entities should pay attention to, such as the issue of medications and the issue of how to best communicate with patients. But instituting other attributes requires resources that may be beyond the reach of the small groups.

No one has discussed how to reach out and educate physicians about becoming more health literate, Hoverman said. What is the plan for this? Might one work with medical societies and associations? Furthermore, she added, the pharmacy aspect is incredibly challenging, particularly when patients use mail order to get their prescriptions. How does one have a conversation about medications when they just appear in a patient's mail box? Another thing that seems to be missing is how to measure the outcomes of one's efforts to become more health literate.

Isham suggested several mechanisms might be used to transmit ideas and to give physicians and others incentives to pursue activities to become more health literate. These mechanisms include quality-improvement organizations,[1] regional quality-improvement collaboratives, requirements instituted by the Centers for Medicare and Medicaid Services (CMS), medical societies, and certifying organizations.

Townzen said that the paper had inspired him. He was happy to see that the changes that Wal-Mart Stores are making, such as reconstructing the counseling queue, fit well with the goal of becoming more health literate. The new system under development will not only provide access to a patient's information at the point of sale or at the register, but it also will provide the right questions to ask the customer to make sure he or she understands. Having the attributes in hand will assist in the development phase. Townzen said that he would like to see some kind of quality check emerge from the paper and the discussion. Are the innovations being

[1] "A Quality Improvement Organization (QIO) consists of groups of doctors and health care experts to check on and improve the care given to people with Medicare." Many QIOs also contract with private companies to conduct reviews of care. https://questions.medicare.gov/app/answers/detail/a_id/1943/~/what-is-a-medicare-quality-improvement-organization-(qio)%3F (accessed January 25, 2012).

developed as good as they think they are? How can the quality of these innovations be measured?

Roundtable member Yolanda Partida asked whether there are opportunities to raise awareness about better choices among one's patients—for example, about a good diet for individuals with diabetes.

Townzen said, yes, absolutely. Walmart is, for example, working with different manufacturers to identify in the stores certain food groups that are better for a diabetic customer, perhaps by installing appropriate signage. And perhaps the pharmacy could direct a patient picking up a prescription for diabetes treatment to the area with those healthful foods.

Hoverman said that in terms of community involvement there are limits to what a small group can do, but larger groups have tremendous opportunities. For example, Walmart has introduced organic foods in its stores and has been able to support some businesses that probably would have gone out of existence without that support. That is a powerful thing for promoting health.

Roundtable member Will Ross noted that both speakers had mentioned financial limitations to implementing the attributes and asked Hoverman to address the issue of return on investment. Hoverman responded that if patients understand their health problems and disease processes, they have a better chance of understanding why they need to take their medications and adhere to a treatment regimen. Therefore they are less likely to be ill, and a visit to the physician's office takes less time. This may take time initially, and there may be many return visits before one begins to see change, but, ultimately, patients have better health. That is a good return on investment.

Schillinger said that return on investment can also be calculated in terms of provider satisfaction, provider retention, and prevention of burnout. The cost of training, recruiting, and hiring needs to be quantified and included in the assessment of a health literate health care organization.

Myra Kline, an audience member from Tulane University, said that she practices in the clinical setting of what used to be a charity hospital in New Orleans. There are major health literacy issues in post-Katrina New Orleans, many of which are due to the large influx of undocumented immigrants. Walmart is where many patients go because it is affordable. How, she asked, does Walmart provide information to patients who have limited English proficiency? And in the university clinical setting, she added, patients are inundated with a barrage of information from their health plans which requires much time to interpret. How does a private practice handle such issues? she asked Hoverman.

Hoverman said that the practice tries to assist its patients in understanding their health insurance plan. For example, many of the patients in her practice are retirees on Medicare who are now being encouraged by mail and telephone to enter a Medicare health maintenance organization. When patients receive these numerous letters, they do not understand what the letters are saying. The patients bring the information to the practice, which tries to help them understand what their choices might be. This is a definite burden on the practice in terms of time and effort, but it is necessary to assist the patients.

Concerning patients with limited English proficiency, Townzen said that printed monographs can be provided only in English, Spanish, and Canadian French. The software does not exist to provide the prescription label in all the languages needed. And certain laws require English to remain on the label so that it can be easily read in case of emergency, such as the patient being taken to an emergency room. There is just not enough space on a label to include everything in English and in another language as well. Furthermore, one cannot simply convert the English text to another language. There are cultural issues and issues of syntax that need to be addressed. Suggestions for new and better ways to address this issue would be welcome, Townzen said.

5

Reaction Panel 3

DENTAL PRACTICE

William Calnon, D.D.S.
Private Practice General Dentistry

Calnon described his practice as a three-person dental practice in Rochester, New York, which has a broad based group of patients. He is also president of the American Dental Association (ADA),[1] which represents 7 out of 10 dentists in this country and, Calnon said, can be viewed as a conduit through which information and education can be provided to dental practitioners in the United States.

One of the attributes listed in the commissioned paper is "Establishing and promoting health literacy as an organizational responsibility." The ADA has done just that, Calnon said. Its Council on Access, Prevention and Interprofessional Relations has as part of its mission to promote community outreach, cultural competency, and health literacy. The council and its advisory committee, the ADA National Advisory Committee on Health Literacy in Dentistry, developed the Health Literacy in Dentistry Action Plan.[2] This is a 5-year plan that focuses on health literacy educa-

[1] The views presented here may not necessarily reflect the policies of the American Dental Association.

[2] The plan can be found at http://ada.org/sections/professionalResources/pdfs/topics_access_health_literacy_dentistry.pdf.

tion and training, advocacy, research, dental practice, and building and maintaining coalitions.

Another activity of ADA is the National Roundtable for Dental Collaboration. It has representation from all types of organizations that are involved with the profession of dentistry, including industry partners and vendors. The group decided to focus on oral health literacy and is working with the Ad Council on a 3-year oral-health literacy campaign, with ADA contributing $1 million of the campaign's total cost of $3.2 million. Another potential partner for work in oral health literacy is Scholastic Publishing. It works on literacy issues through its Read and Rise[3] program, and it is interested in developing an oral health component for its programs, Calnon said.

Other attributes from the commissioned paper that might be of interest to those in dental practice are concerned with inquiry, innovation, and evaluation and with measurement and assessment. A major activity of the ADA is conducting baseline surveys of its members on communication techniques. The National Advisory Committee on Health Literacy in Dentistry is examining the challenges to implementing health literacy practices and is reviewing research on health literacy. A review of printed educational materials, continuing education for dental team members, and other resources is also under way.

Preparing an effective workforce and improving system navigation are other priority attributes for the ADA. There is a pilot program at the schools of dentistry at Temple University and at the University of Oklahoma that is testing a potential new member of dental teams called a community dental health coordinator.[4] Such a coordinator would be, essentially, a patient navigator who would be working directly in communities to help with outreach in oral health literacy. The program is intended to be community-based and culturally and linguistically responsive and to establish linkages with local dental clinics.

Yet another attribute of interest to the ADA is health information technology, Calnon said. The ADA is looking at ways that technology can be used to increase educational effectiveness.

Some of the other attributes listed in the paper are of lower priority for dental providers. Medication safety and communication are not as important for dental providers, for instance, as dentists in private practice tend not to prescribe many medications, mainly just antibiotics and

---

[3] "Read and Rise is a sustainable and systematic literacy engagement program designed to bring families, schools, and communities together to support children's literacy development, while celebrating the positive impact of family culture and tradition." http://www.scholastic.com/aboutscholastic/communityreadandrise.htm (accessed January 25, 2012).

[4] Information about the community dental health coordinator can be found at http://www.ada.org/cdhc.aspx.

analgesics. The bottom line, Calnon said, is that dentists and the ADA are committed to prevention and that oral health literacy and literacy in general are the basis of that preventive work.

HOME HEALTH

Cynthia D. Horton
Visiting Nurses Association of El Paso

The Visiting Nurses Association of El Paso, established in 1967, is a not-for-profit organization that serves about 90 percent of the charitable care provided to the uninsured, homebound people in the community. About 70 percent of that community is Hispanic, Horton said. The core function of the agency is to work with people in their homes and connect them to community resources. The agency is a full-service home health agency with several different core businesses, including hospice, home health, and a private duty side which is private pay. All of these services are provided in the home. But "home" can mean different things, Horton noted, including a rescue mission or a Salvation Army shelter.

A top priority for Horton's agency is to provide culturally relevant education materials. A mandatory component of home health care is teaching. In order to provide home care there must be someone in the home who can take over that care. If the agency cannot find someone to help with self management, a situation that would put the patient at risk, then in extreme cases Adult Protective Services (APS) must be called. Rather than call APS, the agency wants to empower its patients to take over their own care.

A majority of people in the indigent-care program are Spanish speakers, and many are undocumented. Because they are uninsured they wait a long time before deciding to seek medical care. As a result, their conditions are often more acute, and they frequently require hospitalization, but because they are uninsured they are quickly moved out of the hospital, even if they are still very sick. Under these circumstances, a hospital discharge planner calls the agency to let it know that there is an uninsured patient being discharged who needs assistance.

Horton offered an example of what the agency does. There was a construction worker in his thirties who was married with three children and who lived on the outskirts of El Paso. He had a sore on his finger. He saw the sore, put some antibiotic ointment on it, wrapped it with a bandage, and went back to work. This continued for about 8 weeks, with the sore progressively worsening until someone told him he needed to have it examined by a physician.

There is a small clinic on the outskirts of town, the last building on the waterline for the county. This worker lived beyond that. He went to the clinic, which serves about 4,000 people a year who have no other source of care. Most of those served are without running water. The clinic discovered that the worker had Stage 4 melanoma. The clinic then called the agency asking for help. The agency sent a social worker and a nurse to his small mobile home to assess his needs. They found that he required hospice care and reported that to Horton, whose job it is to find what he needs and get it to him.

Because the worker was incontinent and it was becoming unhealthy for him to stay in the same bedroom with his wife, it was decided to obtain a hospital bed for him. The worker's three children were sleeping where the laundry hookups were. It was vital to get him out of that situation. But his mobile home was so small that when the company arrived with the bed they could not fit it through the hallways. There was just no room.

The intervention could not be provided in the home and the hospital would not take him back because he was uninsured and terminal. The agency contacted a partner, the Habitat for Humanity, which has a partnership with a group called Modular Homes. That group put a modular home on his site at no charge so that he could die in peace at home. These are the kinds of problems the agency is faced with and the kinds of strategies it must employ.

Is the agency likely to undertake activities to implement the attributes in the commissioned paper? Yes, absolutely. One activity the agency is undertaking is the development of a user-friendly information technology system that will permit the tracking of patients as they move from program to program, integrating all the services they need.

Another activity concerns communication and building trust. Many of the patients seen by the agency delay visiting a physician and instead self-medicate using remedies that a relative brought back from across the border. Some of these remedies are herbal, and others are items that are over-the-counter drugs in Mexico but prescription medications in the United States (e.g., hydrocodone). Because of the difference, when the patient does see a medical provider he or she generally does not tell the provider about using these medications. Therefore it is important for the agency to communicate with the patient in a way that is comfortable and culturally appropriate so that it can learn about such medication use. It is also important to create trust, to let the patients know that the agency is not going to turn them over to the Immigration and Naturalization Service.

The agency is also planning to undertake company-wide training about health literacy, using the commissioned paper as a base, Horton said.

A major challenge is that despite a high need for community resources, there is a lack of funding which interferes with providing those resources. To try to overcome the lack of direct funding, the agency partners with other organizations whenever possible. For example, the local diabetes association has developed excellent printed materials, and the agency uses those materials rather than expending resources to develop new ones. Progress is being made in the areas of congestive heart failure, diabetes awareness, comprehensive cancer care, and a community-wide falls prevention program. The agency has worked with the community and with experts in the field to find culturally relevant materials and approaches in multiple languages.

The major incentive to become a health literate organization is the people served, Horton said. The better one is able to communicate and provide relevant, culturally appropriate services and materials, the better it will be for the patients. And the agency is also committed to providing not only medical services, but if a family needs food or needs electricity, the agency will work to provide those things. A family that needs food or is worried about losing electricity is too distracted to listen to a nurse describing how to change bandages or engage in a particular therapy.

Horton concluded by saying that two statements in the commissioned paper were particularly relevant for her. One is that a health literate organization views linking patients and social resources as a fundamental part of providing medical care and ensures there are systems in place to make these connections. The other is that comprehension cannot be assumed to be achieved unless it can be demonstrated.

DISCUSSION

Roundtable member Patrick McGarry asked Horton whether a home assessment includes an assessment of the level of literacy and the amount of reading materials in the home. Horton said that the assessment involves a number of things, including the role of all the members of the household, their reading levels, and their food risks.

Roundtable member Winston Wong asked Calnon how the ADA will assess the efficacy of the campaign it is conducting in conjunction with the Ad Council. Are there metrics it will use that are associated with patient engagement or the level of prevention or visits for prevention? Calnon responded that members of the organization are working very closely with the Ad Council in this area because too often outcomes are not assessed. The majority of dental disease is preventable, and the campaign is focusing on changing behavior so that prevention of dental problems is paramount.

Roundtable member Benard Dryer asked Calnon what the role of state health departments and other health organizations should be in promoting understanding about oral health literacy. Calnon responded that all too often professional associations work independently of state dental directors. That should not be the case. Partnerships are needed, particularly in this time of limited resources.

Will Ross, roundtable member, asked both Horton and Calnon about whether patient navigators or community health workers could be used in their organizations' efforts. Horton responded that her agency does use community health workers, or *promotores*, to deliver health information in the community. Everyone has a role to play, so the best approach is to discover each person's passion and figure out how to channel that into community service.

Calnon said that there are enough dentists but that they are not distributed evenly. There are many places in the country that do not have a dental practice. Dental schools have begun to give some preference to individuals from underserved areas with the idea that they might return and practice in those areas. Individuals from a community can assist patients to navigate the system and to be ready to accept dental care. Dental extenders might also play a role. Calnon explained that such individuals, if properly trained and supervised, could provide basic dental care, leaving the more surgical practice to be performed by a trained dentist.

Roundtable member Leonard Epstein asked Horton whether the Visiting Nurses of El Paso work with the community health centers funded by the federal Health Resources and Services Administration. Horton said that they do and that they also work with migrant health programs and the U.S./Mexico Border Commission.

Roundtable member Susan Pisano asked both Horton and Calnon to describe the most persuasive health literacy argument one could make to the leadership of their organizations. Horton said the most persuasive argument is that literacy is not just educational, it is cultural. If one is talking to a patient about diabetes, that patient is running the information through his or her own filter. Developing a health literate organization means identifying the cultural factors and linguistic factors that interfere with or facilitate what patients understand so that information and services are delivered in ways that patients can understand and identify with.

Calnon said that providers need to take into consideration the fact that different patients will hear things differently. Because the outcome sought is better health, it is vital that patients understand what needs to be done. If dentists know that a particular preventive strategy works, it is their duty to educate the public about that strategy.

6

Reaction Panel 4

HEALTH LITERACY AND PATIENT-CENTERED CARE

Ana Pujols-McKee, M.D.
The Joint Commission

McKee began her presentation with an anecdote that illustrates how health literacy challenges can be hidden. She was engaged in a telephone conversation with a man who is in his nineties, and she happened to ask, "What are you doing?" The man laughed and responded that he was trying to file something but that he had forgotten the alphabet. Had she not asked what the man was doing when she called, she would not have realized that he was struggling.

The Joint Commission, McKee said, accredits and certifies 19,000 organizations and programs throughout the United States, including hospitals, homecare, nursing homes, and ambulatory health care facilities. The purpose of the accreditation process is to ensure safety and improve outcomes within the organization. The Joint Commission has had experience with health literacy as far back as 2002 when it, in conjunction with the Centers for Medicare and Medicaid Services (CMS), launched the national Speak Up™ campaign.[1] Other efforts have included the following:

[1] "In March 2002, The Joint Commission, together with the Centers for Medicare and Medicaid Services, launched a national campaign to urge patients to take a role in preventing health care errors by becoming active, involved, and informed participants on the health

- *Hospitals, Language, and Culture: A Snapshot of the Nation* (2004)
- *What Did the Doctor Say?: Improving Health Literacy to Protect Patient Safety* (2007)
- *Exploring Cultural and Linguistic Services in the Nation's Hospitals: A Report of Findings* (2007)
- *One Size Does Not Fit All: Meeting the Health Care Needs of Diverse Populations* (2008)
- Approval of new standards for patient-centered communication (2009)
- *Advancing Effective Communication, Cultural Competence, and Patient- and Family-Centered Care: A Roadmap for Hospitals* (2010)
- Health Equity Advisory Group—internal to the Joint Commission and supported by a grant from the California Endowment

More recently, the Joint Commission has expanded its scope from health literacy to include effective communication, cultural competencies, and patient- and family-centered care. Effective communication is viewed as a two-way process, where messages are negotiated until information is fully understood by both parties. Cultural competency values diversity and assessments, manages the dynamics of difference, and adapts to diversity. Patient- and family-centered care is an innovative approach to planning, delivering, and evaluating health care. In providing such care organizations establish mutually beneficial partnerships with providers, families, and patients, of all ages.

Joint Commission standards are principles that are based on concepts which drive patient safety, process improvement, and protection of patient rights. For every standard, there are elements of performance that an organization must demonstrate. Four key areas of standards are applicable to the attributes of a health literate organization described in the paper, McKee said: leadership, human resources or workforce, provision of care, and the rights and responsibilities of individuals.

The standards related to leadership are focused on making sure that the mission, vision, and goals of the hospital support the safety and quality of care, treatment, and services. The more one focuses on concerns of patient safety, the more likely patient safety will capture the attention, imagination, and innovation of the organization's leadership. Another element of leadership is ensuring that patients with comparable needs receive the same standard of care, treatment, and services throughout the organization.

---

care team. The program features brochures, posters, and buttons on a variety of patient safety topics." http://www.jointcommission.org/facts_about_speak_up_initiatives/ (accessed February 4, 2012).

A second area of standards relevant to attributes of health literacy are the human resources standards. The Joint Commission allows the organization to define the qualifications of its staff. That means there is an opportunity, if the organization wishes, to include education in health literacy as a qualification. Staff do participate in ongoing education and training, some of which is required on an annual basis, and this is another area where health literacy could be included. Finally, staff are evaluated to ensure that they are competent to perform their responsibilities. Health literacy could be included here as well.

The third area in which health literacy can be found in the Joint Commission Standards is in the standards that define provision of care. The hospital is expected to provide assessesments and reassessments of all patients. Some of this may be especially pertinent to health literacy, for example, if nurses are asked to assess a patient's learning preferences. There are many opportunities within this standard of assessment to identify issues of health literaacy. The hospital is also expected to provide education and training, based on each patient's needs and abilitities. One of the elements of performance for this standard is that every patient should identify his or her needs, which could potentially include issues of health literacy.

The fourth area of standards concerns the rights and responsibilities of individuals. A hospital must honor the patient's right to give or withold informed consent. However, if one were to closely examine the informed consent process, one might find that many patients do not understand what they are being told. Some of this is due to the way in which information is presented, some is due to time constraints that foster quick interaction, and some is due to the fact that the time at which the discussion is taking place is a very emotional time for the patient.

A new Joint Commission requirement attempts to address some of these issues by calling for patient-centered communication, bilateral communication, or negotiating information until both parties understand fully. The expanded standards now allow a family member, friend, or other individual to be present with the patient for emotional support during the course of the patient's stay. There is also a requirement that the hospital provide language interpretation and translation services.

The Joint Commission has published a document titled *Advancing Effective Communication, Cultural Competence, and Patient- and Family-Centered Care: A Roadmap for Hospitals*. One chapter provides a checklist on how to assess an organization's readiness to make the kinds of cultural changes and competency changes that improve health literacy in the organization, including the ability to use data in an effective way and the readiness of the leadership and the workforce.

McKee said two attributes were most important. The first is "Promoting health literacy as an organization's responsibility." When an organization's leadership is able to recognize a failure in communication with a patient as a system failure, that is a very sophisticated organization. But it probably also means that the organization has a culture of safety well embedded throughout.

The second key attribute is the one that involves identifying high-risk treatments and transitions. Relevant to this is the area of informed consent discussed earlier. Improving health literacy capabilities in this area offers a tremendous opportunity to improve safety.

All of the attributes should be integrated into the operational functions of the organization—into patient safety initiatives, into patient experience initiatives, and into intiatives that involve community outreach or employee engagement.

Those attributes that are potentially unfeasible are the ones that require rich resources. Until there is information about the return on investment for health literacy interventions, it will be difficult to convince organizations, particularly those that are stuggling financially, that it is valuable and important to move forward in those areas.

The Joint Commission is developing a method of evaluation called the Tracer Method. Such a method will trace a patient's journey throughout the organization, from the point of admission or the emergency room to the patient discharge. In this world of important transitions of care, it is recognized that the tracer must also extend into the patient's home, with homecare, or into the long-term care facility. Evaluating an organization's ability to communicate confidently with the patients would be a component in that tracer method.

It is the vision of the Joint Commission that all people, regardless of their level of education, their ability to read, or their ability to understand English should always experience the safest, highest-quality, best-value health care across all settings. That statement is relevant to what makes an organization health literate, McKee said.

AN EMPLOYER'S VIEW

John Neuberger
QuadGraphics

QuadGraphics was founded in 1971 and is the second largest printer in the Western Hemisphere, Neuberger said. It has 28,000 employees in 80 facilities in North America, Latin America, and Europe. In the United States the facilities are located in very different kinds of areas—some very large and urban, others small and rural—and language issues arise in many areas. About 20 years ago QuadGraphics started providing medical care to its employees, including

- primary care clinics with selected subpecialties;
- wellness and preventive medicine programs;
- an occupational medicince program;
- onsite rehabilitation clinics;
- full-services laboratories, X-rays, pharmacies, and dental services;
- third-party benefit administration and utilitzation review;
- robust information systems; and
- telemedicine.

Health literacy is a cornerstone of a successful health care model, Neuberger said. QuadGraphics, as is the case with any employer, needs a healthy and productive workforce that works every day if the company is to remain competitive in a very competitive market. The organization is also concerned about population health for the 50,000 lives covered under its health plan. If the consumers of care are not health literate, it will cost both the company and the patient money. Health literacy is not just an expense, it is an investment. The indirect costs of poor health literacy include low productivity, absenteeism, presenteeism,[2] and increased workers compensation claims. The company sees health literacy as one of the cornerstones of managing costs, health, and wellness in consumer-driven care.

Of the eighteen attributes discussed in the commissioned paper, several are important to an employer such as QuadGraphics. One is "Provide an infrastructure to avail frontline providers with educational supports and resources." It is important to have have reinforcements at the point of service for what the provider (e.g., the physician, the dentist, the pharmacist, or the physical therapist) has just told the patient. It is not enough just to provide a brochure. It is important to work with the patient to be sure that both patient and provider understand the issues involved in care and agree on what needs to be done to take care of the condition. In the company's clinics 30 minutes per provider is allowed for each visit. The company is willing to pay for this because it believes that allowing that amount of time is effective in promoting health. It provides time for the patient to focus not only on their ailment, but on prevention and wellness issues, such as losing weight, stopping smoking, and family problems.

---

[2] Presenteeism is "the measure of lost productivity cost due to employees actually showing up for work, but not being fully engaged and productive mainly because of personal health and life issue distractions." http://ezinearticles.com/?Presenteeism:-The-Hidden-Costs-of-Business&id=40408 (accessed February 5, 2012).

While interaction at the time of service is key, it is also important for the patient to leave with appropriate written materials or a website reference that reinforces the information exchanged between provider and patient. Even if the patient understands the information at the time of the visit, it is likely that memory and understanding will fade with time. Reinforcement of information is especially important for patients with chronic conditions that need to continue to be managed.

Another important attribute is "Fosters an augmented and prepared workforce to promote health literacy." From the company's perspective this means the presence of integrated health teams to support the provider, including reception staff, the nurse, or others that work in the setting. These staff need to be trained in health literacy and to be sensitive to and understanding of the patient's needs. With such a team the provider can refer the patient to the appropriate staff for continued support—to the dietician to talk about diet, the hygienist to discuss dental care, or the receptionist to make the call to set up needed tests.

The team should reflect the socio-demographic profiles of the population. Members should be prepared to translate the provider's directions into language that the patient understands, to check on understanding and comprehension, to encourage questioning, and to focus on actionable information.

Another important attribute is to "Make health plan and health insurance products more transparent." During open enrollment employees are being asked to make tough choices. They need clear and plain communication. Before any vendor can send information to its employees, Quad-Graphics must first review it to make sure it is understandable for the population served. Plan descriptions need to be made more comprehensible so that families choose the right plan for themselves. The company counsels employees who are having difficulty understanding which plan to choose. Employers have a major role to play in health literacy. They need to engage the employee all year, not just at the time of enrollment, and to encourage employees to take resonsibility for their personal health.

"Make systems more navigable for families working through the health care system" is another important attribute for employers. There are huge challenges in attemping to navigate the complicated and fragmented health care environment. Patients need to feel comfortable asking for help.

There are major challenges to implementing policies and programs aimed at becoming a more health literate organization, Neuberger said. There are no immediate financial incentives for health care organizations. Are health care providers really interested in reducing utilization of services under the current fee-for-service basis? Are they serious about reducing emergency room visits, testing, and so on?

Information needs to be easily accessible to employees. QuadGraphics is in the process of creating a webpage that will provide employees with a variety of information related to their health benefits, including medical and pharmacy benefits, flexible spending accounts, and claims information. With such a page employees will no longer have to navigate multiple sites in order to obtain needed information. Employers also need to develop an advocacy role so as to assist patients in choosing and navigating their health plans. Furthermore, employers can assure that all health care materials are properly geared to various populations. That is what QuadGraphics is doing—making sure that the information is relevant to its different populations of employees. Employers have the financial incentives to ensure that their populations are literate and can navigate the health care system.

Employers are willing to work with providers in their communities in order to create healthier populations. For example, there is one small clinic in one of the QuadGraphic communities that wants to become a medical home. To do so requires a nurse care manager to, among other things, monitor patients. But the clinic cannot pay for a full-time care manager. So the clinic approached QuadGrahics asking if the company would be willing to pay half the salary, and it appears that the company will do this because it is a good investment in employee health.

Neuberger concluded by saying that employers are incentivized and can be partners in working with health care organizations to become more health literate. Employers are willing to pay for better outcomes and better care. However, it is important to have a system for documenting improvements—a system that can monitor patients' understanding of their medical conditions and provide information to develop better practices in order to improve outcomes through improved health literacy.

THE CENTERS FOR MEDICARE AND MEDICAID SERVICES (CMS) PERSPECTIVE

Shari Ling, M.D.
Office of Clinical Standards and Quality

Health literacy is an important topic at a critical time when the country is facing limited resources, Ling said. All of the attributes discussed in the paper are important. They speak to different parts of the system and different issues. Rather than discuss individual attributes separately, Ling bundled them into a few categories and said she thought that it may be worth considering the bundles in terms of what can be done immediately using existing resources versus what requires more long-term solutions. One could also think about them in terms of what is actionable rather than what is ideal. Finally, perhaps those attributes that require health system redesign could be reframed in terms of what can be accomplished or achieved without a complete redesign—that is, what can be tackled now.

The first of the attributes that is critically important—"Promoting health literacy as an organizational responsibility"—falls into the bundle of culture change and the acknowledgment that culture matters. Culture matters for the patients and for the families; it is the filter through which all information flows. This attribute is fundamental but is also the greatest challenge. Other attributes in this bundle include the following:

- Encourage active inquiry, innovation, evaluation, and improvements.
- Encourage and expect question asking.
- Assess the communication climate.
- Recognize and overcome communication barriers.
- Target population health literacy advisory group.

Another important bundle of attributes relates to attention to content. This is particularly crucial in the area of medication safety and communication about medication safety. Conversations around this issue must balance the risks versus the benefits of the recommended interventions. That conversation is dependent upon the patient understanding and believing what is being said, and understanding requires health literacy.

Infrastructure is another important bundle of attributes. There are long-term and short-term infrastructure requirements. "Provider, patient, and family technical assistance" could be provided immediately by offering educational materials that can actually be read and understood. "Enhancing health care system navigability," particularly across transitions, could be addressed in the short term. Longer-term infrastructure requirements include "Leveraging health information technology," "Providing personal health records," and, again, "Enhancing health care system navigability."

In an earlier presentation, Darren Townzen had offered a surprising but informative piece of information when he said that even when personal health records are available, they are not necessarily used. What can be done to make them usable? That is a longer term effort that needs to be undertaken, Ling said.

The final bundle of attributes relates to developing needed skills and tools for the workforce, the individual, and the community. There is an opportunity for private and public partnerships to develop and apply techniques that are never taught in medical school, for example, techniques that are based on learning theories. What motivates an individual to learn? How can understanding this motivation be applied in the medical setting? What lessons can be learned by both providers and patients? The bundle includes the following attributes:

- Assess and track patient comprehension, skills, and problem solving.
- Community resource awareness.
- Provider, patients, and family education resources.
- Promoting health plan and insurance transparency and comprehensibility—access and use.
- Curricula and threshold for health skills.

There are a number of implementation challenges. What will encourage corporations and the health care system to embrace the idea of improving health literacy? From the perspective of the CMS, this requires an evidence base. It also requies acknowledging that perception and perspective matter: A message has to be perceived and understood in order to be acted upon. At a system level it must be recognized that there are burdens on the providers and the system. A provider has a specified number of minutes to collect a patient history, conduct the examination, and develop a plan with recommendations. And this is true even in a system that has powerful electronic health records. Resources are a huge challenge. How can these interventions be paid for? And finally, policy change requires due process. Organizations are usually slow to change. Stakeholder and public engagement and input are critical.

Encouraging the implementation of the attributes starts with a vision and requires both strategy and resources. CMS is a major force and a trustworthy partner for the continued improvement of health and health care for all Americans, Ling said. Figure 6-1 ilustrates the "three-part aim" of CMS. At the center are the patient and the family, which means that the challenge of achieving health literacy is itself at the center.

As for strategy, there is no "silver bullet," Ling said. Many incentives are needed to change behavior. Changing patient behavior relies on literacy, on comprehension, and on understanding. Changing provider behavior has a different set of challenges, but theories of behavioral intervention apply there, too. Intensive support must be offered for the painstaking work needed to improve.

Figure 6-2 shows the various implementation levers for change. This slide has been presented before with quality at the center, but the concepts apply equally well with health literacy at the center. There are numerous opportunities. The conditions of participation, or COP, can be seen at the bottom of the diagram. CMS writes conditions of participation for all providers. If they want to participate, they must abide by the rules. Perhaps the COP offers an opportunity for encouraging the attributes.

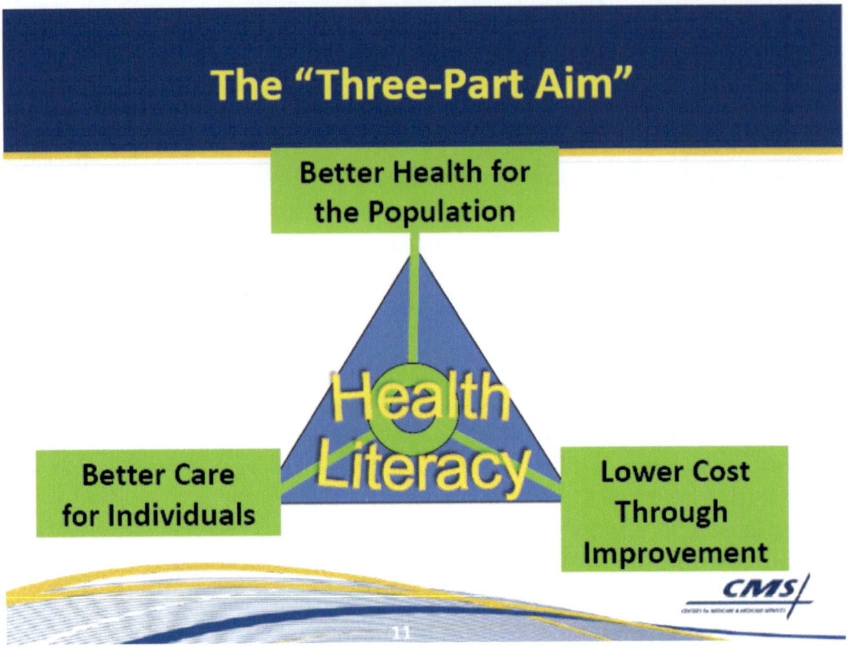
The "Three-Part Aim"
Better Health for the Population
Health Literacy
Better Care for Individuals
Lower Cost Through Improvement
CMS

FIGURE 6-1 Three part aim.
SOURCE: Ling, 2011.

Quality-improvement organizations are a potential lever for observing, studying, planning, and demonstrating improvement, and public acknowlegment of a job well done can provide incentive. Existing quality-improvement sites include Hospital Compare, Home Health Compare, ESRD (End Stage Renal Disease) Compare, and Physician Compare. Perhaps aspects of what matters in health literacy can be integrated into the quality measurement and reporting schemes in these organizations. Can some of the concepts embodied in these attributes, for example, be extracted from the electronic health record in order to support a quality measure construct? If so, that would support an operational and implementation strategy.

Patient safety is another avenue for incentives. Perhaps some of the attributes could be integrated into the patient safety data formats offered by the Agency for Healthcare Research and Quality. Other projects include improving health literacy as a key component. Partnership for Patients, which is focused on reducing hospital readmissions, is predicated on the idea that such reductions can be achieved with increased patient understanding and comprehension. The CMS diabetes disparities project

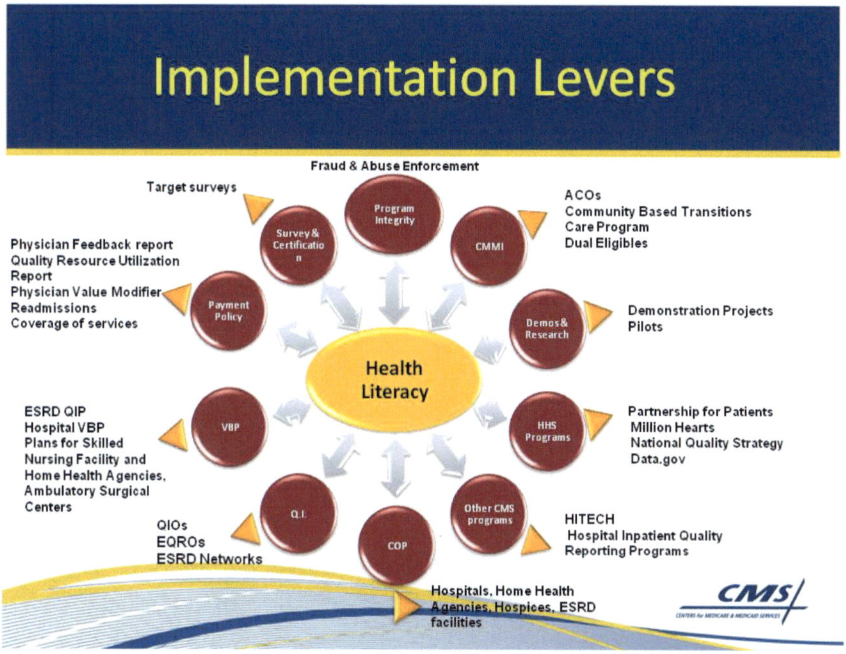

FIGURE 6–2 Implementation levers.
NOTE: Acronyms are as follows: ACOs are accountable care organizations; ARRA is the American Recovery and Reinvestment Act; ASC VBP is ambulatory surgical center value-based purchasing; CAH VBP is critical access hospital value-based purchasing; EQROs are external quality review organizations; ESRD is End-stage Renal Disease; ESRD QIP is End-stage Renal Disease quality incentive program; HH is home health; HITECH is the Health Information Technology for Economic and Clinical Health Act; IQR is inpatient quality reporting; IRF is inpatient rehabilitation facility; LTCH is long term care hospital; OQR is outpatient quality reporting; PRQS is physician quality reporting system; QIOs are quality improvement organizations; SNF is skilled nursing facility; and VBP is value-based purchasing.
SOURCE: Ling, 2011.

addresses cultural competency and improving health literacy through better communication with Medicare beneficiaries in minority and underserved populations.

Ling concluded her presentation by saying that the attributes discussed in the commissioned paper provide an opportunity for moving the important health literacy agenda forward.

DISCUSSION

Roundtable member Benard Dreyer said that his hospital was recently surveyed by the Joint Commission. During the week that the surveyors spent in the hopsital, not once did anyone ask about anything related to health literacy or health communication, even though they asked about many other specific things. Unless the importance of health literacy is made explicit, he said, hospitals will not pursue it. Because hopsitals are under a variety of pressures, they are only going to respond to those who regulate or pay them. Those are the pressures that create change. How can health literacy be made explicit in the ways that CMS regulates and that the Joint Commission accredits health care organizations?

McKee said that the Joint Commission must achieve a balance between being too prescriptive and too nondirectional. One opportunity is provided by surveyor education and the need for a specific focus on health literacy training. The training should address not only what to look for and discuss with hospital staff, but also what to look for and discuss with patients.

Ling said that health literacy must be spoken about, particularly within the area of care transitions and patient safety. An actionable opportunity for CMS would be to examine its disparities data and to approach health literacy through its quality-improvement efforts.

Roundtable member Will Ross said that the relationship of health literacy to quality was not emphasized in the figure of implementation levers (Figure 6-2). Yet that is what health literacy is about—improving quality. Perhaps the discussion should be reframed, he said. George Isham, the roundtable chair, added that the figure is useful because it provides a guide to potential points of action or influence. Another action pathway to add to the figure would be access to health information technology and other resources for small private practices.

Ling said that the figure is meant to provide a framework of opportunities to think about. Reaching individual physicians and providers is challenging. Avenues in the past have included educational sessions in the context of the physician quality reporting program and electronic health record incentives. Operational health literacy definitions and action items would help tremendously.

Roundtable member Cindy Brach said that employers are important players in encouraging health literate practices and that their purchasing power offers them levels by which change can be encouraged. For example, employers make decisions about which insurance plans to offer and which providers to contract with. How would the attributes discussed in the paper help an employer think about information provided by a health plan and about its health literate practices? For CMS, will the information in the commissioned paper help with developing surveyor training and checklists they might use?

Neuberger agreed that employers do have a major role to play in health literacy. Everyone has a stake in health literacy. Poor health literacy contributes significantly to the cost of care because if patients do not comprehend what they are supposed to do, they don't do it, which results in poorer outcomes and greater costs. QuadGraphics has learned not to use acronyms when explaining health plan options, Neuberger said. Providing incentives for preventive care and wellness programs is another way to influence the options chosen.

Ling said that CMS values the concepts of health literacy. The difficulty comes at the operational level. How can the terms be defined in ways that are measurable? What criteria should be used in determining whether an organization is health literate? Is there a scale that could be used and implemented within one of the quality reporting programs? What are the sources of data? Having a data source would make it easier for CMS to achieve health literacy objectives through the survey process or the quality measurement, reporting, and improvement programs.

Brach said that the Agency for Healthcare Research and Quality has developed a health literacy supplement to the Consumer Assessment of Health Providers Survey.[3] And the agency is about to finalize an HCAHPS (Hospital Consumer Assessment of Healthcare Providers and Systems) health literacy supplement and is currently working on one for health plans as well. Ling replied that these would be wonderful tools to have. Another thing that is needed, she said, is to demonstrate that health literacy interventions support affordability. Perhaps such efforts could be included in the health care innovation challenge.[4]

McKee said that there is opportunity to provide education in health literacy. The Joint Commission has sentinel event alerts that attract a great deal of attention. Health literacy might be a topic for an alert. Furthermore, Joint Commission Resources[5] might expand its scope of services to include health literacy. Another opportunity is to assess health literacy as a potential contributing factor when conducting a sentinel event review

[3] The supplement "focuses on assessing providers' activities to foster and improve the health literacy of patients." https://www.cahps.ahrq.gov/surveys-guidance/item-sets/health literacy.aspx (accessed February 5, 2012).

[4] A new CMS initiative that "will invest up to $1 billion in support of local innovation in communities across the nation to achieve three-part aim outcomes: better care, better health and lower costs through continuous improvement." http://innovations.cms.gov/ (accessed February 5, 2012).

[5] Joint Commission Resources provides education, publications, consultation, and evaluation regarding accreditation, standards development, good practices, and health care quality improvement. http://www.jcrinc.com/About-JCR/ (accessed February 5, 2012).

or a review of any adverse event. One of the services that the Joint Commission provides to its accredited organizations is being able to review a sentinel event with the organization. There is a team of clinicians who dedicate 100 percent of their time to reviewing these events. Communication is the theme that runs through most of the 900 sentinel events reviewed each year. The traditional approach to a review does not get to the granular detail of the communication defect, but rather it defines the issue in general as a problem in communication. In general, the implications of health literacy may not be identified. If communication is the theme, what often occurs is that the patient misunderstood instructions. The defect is then assumed to be the responsibility of the patient, not the organization or the process. McKee said she would examine how these sentinel reviews could include a process that helps identify opportunities with the organizations to address systemic literacy defects.

Roundtable member Yolanda Partida asked Ling whether she thought there was an opportunity for CMS to create incentives for health promotion and health preservation. Ling responded that CMS can implement incentives within the limits of its authority. It can cover conditions and can pay for medical services for Medicare beneficiaries that include an annual wellness visit. Health risk assessment is still evolving. There is an increasing acknowlegment that behavior matters, yet any new thing proposed must go through rule making, which includes a requirement that CMS consider and respond to every comment. That discussion is an opportunity that plays out in a public forum during the course of rule making.

Roundtable member Clarence Pearson asked Neuberger what arguments could be advanced to employers to encourage them to support health literacy in an environment where employees stay with the same company for only 4 or 5 years on average. Neuberger responded that where turnover is very high, it is more difficult to see a postive return on investment (ROI). Yet for many employers wellness is a core strategy. For employers paying the bills, wellness is a much better investment than sickness.

Roundtable member Ruth Parker said that employers are key stakeholders to engage and are incredibly powerful drivers. What about these attributes is most useful in talking with employers? she asked Neuberger. Neuberger responded that over the past few decades health plans have mediated between the providers and the payers. As a result, employers lost the opportunity to talk with each other on a regular basis. But health care issues and costs are now so significant for employers that they are hungry for discussion. They reach out to hospitals and health systems around the country. Often the health care organizations think the entire discussion is about price. And sometimes it is, but more importantly it is about outcomes, about creating and maintaining a healthy workforce. Employers want to talk with those providing the care, to work together to face key issues of improving care and outcomes.

Roundtable member Paul Schyve noted that the workshop discussion on how organizations can become health literate involved three different kinds of influences: the role of extrinsic requirements (such as those from regulators or accreditors), the role of intrinsic motivation, and the role of incentives. From the perspective of the Joint Commission, and probably also of CMS, the preference would be to not hear that an organization is doing something because it is required. These groups would rather receive a thank-you for reminding the organization what needs to be done, for evaluating how well it is doing, and for giving advice about how to do it better because only if there is the intrinsic motivation does one have a high level of success.

Either positive incentives (e.g., more pay) or negative incentives (e.g., less money) can be used to encourage the health literacy agenda. But there are also perverse incentives, that is, putting in place an incentive system that keeps an organization from doing what it intrinsically wishes to do. And that, Schyve said, is a major problem in health care today.

The roundtable fosters discussions aimed at developing intrinsic motivation. CMS and the accrediting bodies create extrinsic requirements. And industry is trying to produce incentives as well, although it also has extrinsic requirements in its contracting terms. But if these incentives continue to operate in separate silos the result will be inefficieny and ineffectiveness. All three things are important—intrinsic motivation, extrinsic requirements, and the incentives. At the same time, working collaboratively is needed in order to align these three influences.

Roundtable member Winston Wong agreed with the points that Schyve made in the discussion about extrinsic and intrinsic incentives. Benard Dreyer, while agreeing with the general discussion of intrinsic and extrinsic incentives, said that there are many organizations that do view health literacy as an intrinsic value, but they are under attack because of limited resources.

REFERENCE

Ling, S. 2011. *Centers for Medicare and Medicaid Services (CMS) Perspective*. Presentation at the Institute of Medicine Workshop on Attributes of a Health Literate Organization, November 16. Washington, DC.

7

Reflections on Lessons Learned

George Isham, the roundtable chair, asked the members of the roundtable to reflect on what they heard and learned from the commissoned paper and the presentations delivered during the workshop.

Paul Schyve said that most of his reflections centered on the subject of implementation. The first issue was the need for interaction among intrinsic motivation, extrinsic requirements, and extrinsic incentives, as discussed earlier. The second concerns what can be done directly with the consumer to increase health literacy in the population. The third is how to enable those providing care to do so in a health literate way.

Winston Wong said it is ironic that in some areas there is no thought of discussing return on investment (ROI), such as with the simple safety precaution of washing hands before seeing a patient. When does health literacy cease to be a question of ROI and instead become basic to providing good care? To move forward requires three things. One is to make the case for system-level reform. Health literacy is not just a personal attribute; it is an issue of system-level change. Second, how can meaningful measures for outcomes of health literacy interventions be developed, both in clinical areas and for population health? Third, instead of talking about incentives, what are the financial models that align with supporting the development of health literacy proficiency?

Patrick McGarry said that the workshop and, in particular, Horton's presentation brought home why health literacy is important—because of people and because their beliefs and the context in which they live affect health. Health literacy interventions take these determinants into account.

Margaret Loveland said that the commissioned paper makes clear the enormous task involved in instilling concepts and practices of health literacy into providers and payors. It is encouraging to hear from the panelists that progress is being made and that some organizations and individuals are beginning to act on health literacy. Another important point that emerged from the paper and the discussion is the idea that health literacy is closely related to patient safety, which may motivate providers to incorporate health literacy into their practices. Finally, although none of the panelists represented the pharmaceutical industry, that sector has been involved in health literacy activities for quite some time because of its recognition that health literacy and medication safety are closely related. Partnerships with that industry may be one way to advance the implementation of health literate practices, she said.

Benard Dreyer expressed great admiration for the commissioned paper and the presentations. He suggested that the 18 attributes described should be reorganized and prioritized in a way that connects them more directly to accountable care organizations or patient-centered medical homes or patient safety. It might also be useful to place them in a Venn diagram with health disparities, he said. Second, something that is specific to children needs to be added. Third, the discussion about the diversity of cultures and language, which is included in the paper, should be elevated to a more prominent discussion. Finally, there is the issue of how to move the discussion into action. One of the points made is that there must be defined measures for assessing whether an organization is health literate. There are a number of current measures, including the new HCAHPS (Hospital Consumer Assessment of Healthcare Providers and Systems), that can be used as a start. Identification and discussion of measures may be a worthy topic for the roundtable to follow up on.

Will Ross said that the paper and presentations effectively married health literacy to dimensions of quality. As a consequence, this has elevated health literacy as a recognized part of the pathway to quality care. The roundtable should begin discussions about and an examination of the relationship between health literacy and quality.

Ruth Parker quoted Oliver Wendell Holmes, Jr., who said, "I would not give a fig for the simplicity on this side of complexity, but I would give my life for the simplicity on the other side of complexity."[1] The paper and the discussion have shown that health literacy is complicated. The next step is to discover how to make the concepts and discussion understandable, clear, actionable, and useful.

Sharon Barrett said that the paper and discussion has helped move the focus from emphasis on the patient's responsibility to be health literate to

[1] Many attribute this quote to Oliver Holmes, Sr.

a focus on the responsibility of the provider and the system to encourage health literate practice. It is important to understand what the return on investment of health literate practice is. Another important concept that emerged is the need to trace what happens to patients across a continuum that includes not only the health care setting but also the patient's cultural and home environments because those environments play key roles in determining whether patients follow treatment regimens.

Clarence Pearson said that the workshop has shown the importance of getting four sectors—government, business, nonprofits, and academia—to work together to foster health literate practices.

Susan Pisano said that the commissioned paper was fabulous and encouraging. The presentations were also encouraging because they showed the commitment of many different kinds of providers and organizations to the concepts of health literacy. It will be important to help organizations translate the paper into action. Leadership will be crucial, but it is important to note that leadership does not have to start at the top of an organization. There have been tremendous grassroots efforts that have culminated with an organization's chief executive officer embracing ideas that began at the bottom of the organization.

Scott Ratzan said the ideas presented in the presentations and the paper were inspiring. Of particular interest, he said, were the things that the American Dental Association has undertaken to improve oral health literacy. Oral health literacy is an area that the roundtable may wish to continue to pursue, in addition to its upcoming workshop on that topic. The paper itself might benefit from an executive summary or a framework for action, he suggested. Is there some way to fit important points on one page so that they will be more accessible to a broader audience? Another issue to explore is a framework for what organizations might do to become health literate. Perhaps one could develop checklists or scorecards that could be used to assess the status toward achieving each of the attributes.

Yolanda Partida noted that the discussion has focused on health care, but when one talks about overall return on investment, one must focus on health, on preservation, and on disease prevention.

Cindy Brach said the commissioned paper was fantastic. The majority of the paper emphasizes the system or the organization. The presentations were also inspiring, but discussion frequently shifted to a focus on increasing the health literacy of patients. It is important not to lose the idea that the system can be health literate.

Martha Gragg said she agreed with one of the speakers that the 18 attributes presented in the paper need to be bundled. Hoverman made the point that she was hearing about some of the tools for health literate practice for the first time. Perhaps the revised paper could include a resource guide. Another point is the need to think about measures—what particular measures are needed and useful and how can these be developed.

An audience member said that there is absolutely a need for showing return on investment for health literacy interventions. Even with organizational champions and leadership, if one cannot show a return on investment, then that investment will not continue. Moving from the elevated discussion down to practicalities, the audience member asked, What are the actionable things that can be done? How can we institutionalize health literacy into our organizations, associations, and agencies?

Cynthia Baur, another audience member, said that the commissioned paper is well aligned with the *National Action Plan to Improve Health Literacy* (ODPHP, 2010). Those developing the plan recognized that it is a challenge to connect strategies or attributes with what one actually does. There is a Centers for Disease Control and Prevention website[2] that has a number of tools and resources for organizations to use. Another point, Baur said, is that from her perspective health literacy encompasses both communication and education. These approaches may require slightly different infrastructures and supports. An example involving tobacco may help clarify this difference. One can deliver a message about the need to stop smoking, and that is a communication activity. It is another level of activity and support to think about supporting someone in the act of quitting smoking. In going forward with the paper, one might think about that idea. How does an organization communicate or deliver messages as well as educate or support behavior change?

Audience member Steven Rush said that UnitedHealth created a survey, based on the national action plan, to audit itself on health literacy. It is an interesting tool and ties in very nicely with the attributes discussed at the workshop.

Leonard Epstein said the commissioned paper has the potential for two major conceptual shifts. The first is, as the title says, to focus on "the other side of the coin," that is, on health literacy at the system level. The other shift is to integrate the concepts of health literacy with cultural language and plain language as essential ingredients for effective communication. The presentations foster support for broadening the concept of health literacy in these ways.

Deborah Fritz suggested a communication strategy. It would be easy, she said, to reframe the paper in terms of what is desirable versus what is affordable. But if framed that way, it is easily dismissed. Rather, as this paper is disseminated, it should be defended as a vision of a health literate organization. Engle's proposed model that biological, psychological,

[2] See http://www.cdc.gov/healthliteracy/.

and social factors all play a significant role in disease or illness[3] was seen as utopian when it was published, but it led to a revolution in thinking about health and medicine. This paper also has the potential to change the way that people think.

George Isham said that the group discussed the need to track a patient across a continuum. There is also a need for integration across a continuum, including the need to integrate dental, medical care, and mental health care. This applies to health literacy as well. The commissioned paper has taken the conversation a long way in terms of practical steps for becoming health literate and the rationale behind those steps. Judging by the number and tenor of the comments during the day, everyone is eager to begin to use the input provided to revise and strengthen the paper.

The first panel identified the major challenge to implementing health literate practices as financing. Isham agreed with Fritz that framing implementation as an issue of resources is a disservice to the importance of health literacy. Health literacy is essential to good patient care. There is an opportunity to think about these attributes in terms of organizational effectiveness, using the concepts that come out of business schools about effective use of resources. Another way to think about these attributes is to think about the concepts in the report *Crossing the Quality Chasm: A New Health System for the 21st Century* (IOM, 2001).

REFERENCES

IOM (Institute of Medicine). 2001. *Crossing the Quality Chasm: A New Health System for the 21st Century*. Washington, DC: National Academy Press.

ODPHP (Office of Disease Prevention and Health Promotion). 2010. *National Action Plan to Improve Health Literacy*. Washington, DC: U.S. Department of Health and Human Services.

[3] George L. Engel at the University of Rochester proposed the biopsychosocial model in 1977 in an issue of *Science*.

Appendix A

The Other Side of the Coin: Attributes of a Health Literate Health Care Organization

Dean Schillinger, M.D.[1]
Debra Keller, M.D., M.P.H.[2]

INTRODUCTION

Background

Health literacy has been defined as "the degree to which individuals have the capacity to obtain, process, and understand basic health information and services needed to make appropriate health decisions" (IOM, 2004). Health literacy encompasses a range of skills that individuals need to function effectively in a complex and demanding health care environment. These include literacy skills (reading and writing), oral skills (listening and speaking), numerical calculation and quantitative interpretation skills (numeracy), and, increasingly, Internet navigation skills. Nearly 90 million adults in the United States have limited health literacy. While limited health literacy affects individuals across the entire spectrum of socio-demographic characteristics, it disproportionally affects more vulnerable populations, including the elderly, disabled individuals, people with lower socioeconomic status, ethnic minorities, those with limited English proficiency, and people with limited education (National Center for Education Statistics, 2006). Some of these subgroups are precisely the

[1] Division of General Internal Medicine and Health Communications Program, Center for Vulnerable Populations, Department of Medicine at San Francisco General Hospital, University of California, San Francisco.
[2] Division of General Internal Medicine, Department of Medicine at San Francisco General Hospital, University of California, San Francisco.

populations that have the potential to benefit the most from the implementation of the Patient Protection and Affordable Care Act (ACA), especially if health literacy barriers are attended to (Martin and Parker, 2011).

Compared to individuals with adequate health literacy, individuals with limited health literacy have been shown to have greater difficulty in communicating with clinicians (Schillinger et al., 2004), to be less likely to participate in shared decision making (Sarkar et al., 2011), and to face greater barriers in managing chronic illnesses (Cavanaugh et al., 2008; Williams et al., 1998). Furthermore, limited health literacy appears to be a barrier to access to care, receipt of preventive and self-management support services, and safe medication management (Sarkar et al., 2008, 2011; Sudore et al., 2006). Compared to populations with adequate health literacy, populations with limited health literacy have been shown to have worse self-reported health (Baker et al., 1997), higher rates of many chronic conditions (Sudore et al., 2006), worse quality of life, and intermediate markers of health in some chronic conditions (Schillinger et al., 2002); to experience serious medication errors (Schillinger et al., 2005); and to have increased risk of hospitalization (Baker et al., 2002) and mortality (Sudore et al., 2006). Compared to patients with adequate health literacy, patients with limited health literacy exhibit patterns of utilization of care reflecting a greater degree of unmet needs, such as excess emergency room visits and hospitalizations, even when comorbid conditions and health insurance status are held constant (Hardie et al., 2011). It has been estimated that limited health literacy leads to excess health expenditures of greater than $100 billion annually (Vernon et al., 2007). Improving limited health literacy has been identified as a key strategy to improving the safety, quality, and value of health care (Joint Commission, 2007; National Quality Forum, 2009).

Rationale for This Paper

The vast majority of research on health literacy has focused on characterizing patients' deficits, on how best to measure a patient's health literacy, and on clarifying relationships between a patient's limited health literacy and health outcomes. In addition, most health literacy intervention research has studied how to intervene with patients who have limited health literacy.

There is a growing appreciation, however, that health literacy is a dynamic state that represents the balance (or imbalance) between (a) an individual's capacities to comprehend and apply health related knowledge to health-related decisions and to acquire health-related skills, and (b) the health literacy–related demands and attributes of the health care system. There is a clear need to develop, in parallel, a set of strategies that health care organizations can develop and implement to enable patients and families to access and benefit as much as possible from the range of health care services and to successfully interact with the range of health care entities involved in contemporary health care. The need to address system-level factors that place undue health literacy demands on all patients utilizing the health care system has been emphasized by a variety of government entities, public policy organizations, trade organizations, and research funders, including the Surgeon General's Office (U.S. Surgeon General, 2006), the American Medical Association Foundation (AMA, 2007a, 2007b), the Joint Commission (Joint Commission, 2007), America's Health Insurance Plans (America's Health Insurance Plans, n.d.), the U.S. Department of Health and Human Services Office of Disease Prevention and Health Promotion (HHS, 2010), the Agency for Healthcare Research and Quality, and the National Institutes of Health.

There is perhaps no more critical time than now to shift focus from the health literacy skills of patients to the health literacy–promoting attributes of health care organizations. Enactment of the Patient Protection and Affordable Care Act (ACA)[3] provides opportunities to improve the experience of care and the health outcomes for limited–health literacy populations through insurance reform, Medicaid expansion, and the establishment of health insurance exchanges. Maximizing this opportunity will require that health care organizations attend to the communication needs of limited–health literacy populations. The success of a number of ACA-related redesign initiatives, such as patient-centered medical homes (PCMHs) and accountable care organizations (ACOs) will depend on the stewardship of health care organizations committed to prioritizing the needs of limited–health literacy populations. The expected benefits of insurance expansion will depend on individuals' ability to navigate the complexities of the insurance exchange; without special assistance and institutional commitments, many individuals may not fully benefit from the new system (Martin and Parker, 2011; Sommers and Epstein, 2010). In addition, through the Health Information Technology for Economic and Clinical Health Act (HITECH Act) legislation created to stimulate the adoption of electronic health records and supportive technology, health care providers are being offered financial incentives for demonstrating meaningful use of electronic health records (EHRs), including sharing detailed health information with patients electronically. Whether the benefits of health information technology (IT) will accrue for patients with the greatest needs for communication support will depend on the uptake of health IT among populations with limited health literacy. This, in turn,

[3] 111th Congress, 2nd session. March 23, 2010. Patient Protection and Affordable Care Act. In Public Law 148.

will depend on the extent of investments made to tailor products to the needs of these populations and the health systems that disproportionately care for them.

This paper attempts to identify and describe a set of goals or attributes that diverse health care organizations can aspire to so as to mitigate the negative consequences of limited health literacy and improve access to and the quality, safety, and value of health care services. We describe organizations that have committed to improving and reengineering themselves as "health literate health care organizations" so as to better accommodate the communication needs of populations with limited health literacy, which reinforces the notion that the health care sector shares significant responsibility in promoting health literacy (IOM, 2004).

A foundational principle of health literate health care organizations is that they make clear and effective patient communication a priority across all levels of the organization and across all communication channels. These organizations recognize that health literacy skills are highly variable among the populations they serve and that many of their systems are poorly designed to take into account limited health literacy skills. They also recognize that literacy, language, and culture are intertwined and, as such, their health literacy efforts complement and augment effort to improve their organizations' linguistic and cultural competencies and capacities. These organizations also recognize that clinician–patient miscommunication is very common, and they apply a "universal precautions" approach to communication, whereby communication is simplified to the greatest extent possible and comprehension is not assumed to be achieved unless it can be demonstrated. "Universal precautions" represents a public health approach to communication that attempts to ensure effective basic communication for the largest proportion of the population at the lowest cost. Health literate health care organizations, however, also pay particular attention to ensuring that patient skill-building efforts reach the populations most in need by making special investments, and they recognize that special system redesign efforts may be needed to further reduce health literacy demands in order to better match the health literacy demands of the health care system with the skills of subpopulations so as to mitigate the untoward effect of individuals' limited health literacy skills on their health. A health literate health care organization that openly acknowledges the centrality of clear and interactive communication and invests in optimizing communication for more vulnerable populations can realize benefits for patient access, satisfaction, quality, and safety; can reduce unnecessary patient suffering and costs; can enhance health care provider well-being; and can improve its risk management profile. Finally, a health literate health care organization recognizes the centrality of interprofessional communication as an important means to reduce the informational demands on patients, especially during transitions in care.

The most proximate goals of these organizational investments are to maximize the extent of patients' and families' capacities to (a) comprehend and engage in recommended preventive health behaviors and receive preventive health care services if desired; (b) recognize changes in health states that require attention and access health care services accordingly; (c) develop meaningful, ongoing relationships with health care providers based on open communication and trust; (d) obtain timely and accurate diagnoses for both acute and chronic health conditions; (e) comprehend the meaning of their illness, their options for treatment, and the anticipated health outcomes; (f) build and refine the skills needed to safely and effectively manage their conditions at home and to communicate with the health care team when illness trajectory changes; (g) report their communication needs or comprehension gaps; (h) make informed health care decisions that reflect their values and wishes; and (i) effectively navigate transitions in care. In addition, these investments can enable people to make more appropriate health care coverage choices based on their own health needs or those of their families, to better comprehend the range of benefits and services available to them and how to access them, and to be more aware of the financial implications of their health care choices so as to improve decision making.

The list of attributes and goals for health literate health care organizations included in this paper is by no means exhaustive, and it simply represents our attempt to synthesize a body of knowledge and practice supported to the greatest extent possible by the state of the science in the young field of health literacy. The attributes and goals that we outline are most well-developed for and most clearly applicable to organizations that provide direct care to patients. However, a majority are also relevant to the broader range of organizations and institutions that comprise the modern health care system, such as health insurers and health plans, pharmacies, pharmacy benefits managers, disease management companies, and vendors of health IT and patient education products. We see this paper less as a definitive response to the challenge of defining a "health literate health care organization" and more as an attempt to advance a vision of how organizations should evolve to be more responsive to the needs of populations with limited health literacy in tangible ways, thereby improving care for all.

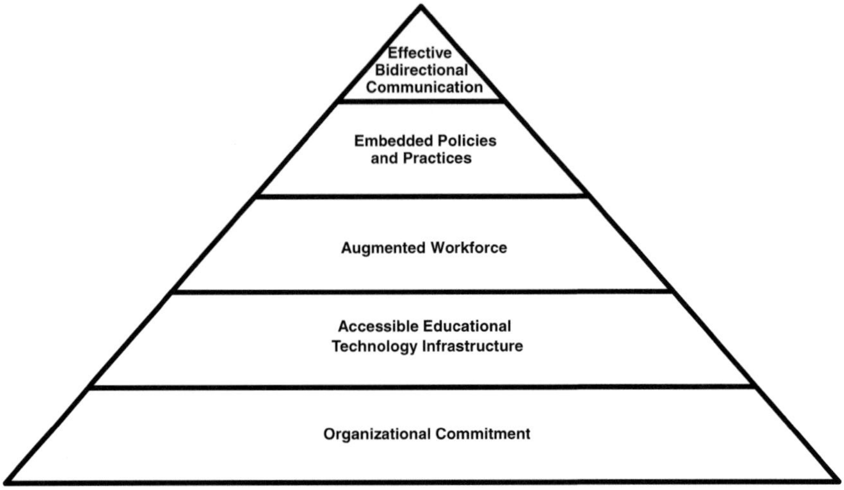

FIGURE A-1 Features of a health literate health care organization.

ATTRIBUTES AND GOALS FOR HEALTH LITERATE HEALTH CARE ORGANIZATIONS

When making communication an organizational priority, health literate health care organizations embrace a package of central principles and practices with respect to organizational structures, processes, personnel, and technologies for enabling patient care and population management so as to mitigate the untoward effect of individuals' limited health literacy skills on their health and health care costs (Figure A-1).

1. Establish Promoting Health Literacy as an Organizational Responsibility

Organizational leaders should establish a culture of clear communication. Leadership should raise organization-wide awareness about the importance of health literacy and clear communications across all facets of the health care system and should participate in local, state, and national efforts to improve organizational responses to limited health literacy. Organizational leaders should make clear statements about the responsibility of all sectors of their health care system to advance patients' and families' capacities to learn about their illness, carry out self-care, effectively communicate, and make informed decisions. Leaders should create an organizational expectation that patients, families, and caregivers are well supported in understanding and managing their health and that suboptimal communication outcomes due to lack of effort, expertise, or infrastructure are viewed as a systems failures and are addressed through systems redesign. Health literate health care organizations may choose to employ a health literacy officer or high-level health literacy task force to ensure that health literacy is deeply, explicitly, and continually integrated into quality-improvement activities, cultural and linguistic competence efforts, patient safety initiatives, and strategic planning. Ongoing organizational assessments should be carried out to reflect organizational performance and progress in promoting health literacy. Promoting health literacy should be considered when planning organizational operations, job descriptions, evaluation metrics, and budgets. Systems can be put in place to ensure that members of the health care team have adequate time and incentives to learn and implement basic health literacy tools as well as to access more sophisticated resources when necessary. Resources can be earmarked for patient education experts and community advisory group members who can both train frontline providers and develop and administer specialized curricula to patients with demonstrated need.

2. Develop a Culture of Active Inquiry, Partner in Innovation, and Invest in Rigorous Evaluations of Operations Improvements

While the untoward health and economic outcomes associated with limited health literacy are now established, the value of existing intervention research to health literacy programming at the operations level is hampered by the relative infancy of the field and inconsistent results. A recent systematic review of interventions designed to mitigate the effects of limited literacy found consistent results for only a select number of discrete design features aimed at improving participant comprehension (presenting essential information by itself or first, presenting information so that the high number is better, presenting numerical information in tables rather than text, adding icon arrays to numerical information, and adding video to verbal narrative) (Sheridan et al., 2011). In addition, some studies found that intensive mixed-strategy interventions focusing on self- and disease-management reduced emergency and hospital utilization as well as disease severity. The common features of mixed-strategy interventions that changed health outcomes included having a basis in theory, carrying out a pilot test, being high intensity, having an emphasis on skill building, and being delivered by a health professional. Finally, the relative paucity of real-world implementation research involving representative populations in nonacademic health care settings has further limited the value of prior research efforts for informing health literacy programming at an organizational level. Rather than waiting for others to identify solutions, health literate health care organizations develop mutually beneficial partnerships with health literacy researchers spanning a range of disciplines to help develop, identify, implement, and evaluate health literacy interventions whose results will have an immediate relevance to organizational processes (Allen et al., 2011).

3. Measure and Assess the Health Literacy Environment and Communication Climate

A health literate health care organization establishes ongoing mechanisms and metrics to measure the success of its system in achieving the health literacy attributes described above, to evaluate special health literacy programs, and to identify areas for further improvement. Such organizations perform institutional health literacy reviews focused on the health literacy environment and the variety of communication and support systems in place. Templates for such reviews have been made available by the Agency for Healthcare Research and Quality (AHRQ) for both health practices (DeWalt et al., 2010) and pharmacies (Jacobson et al., 2007) and can be adjusted to apply to any health care organization. An organizations can undertake a 360-degree assessment of its communication climate and culture. For example, there is evidence that a better organizational communication climate, as measured by the Communication Climate Assessment Tool, is associated with better quality of care (Wynia et al., 2010). In addition, if investments have been made for the educational support infrastructure as described above, organizations can monitor patient understanding of their medical conditions both on individual and population levels. Organizations can also track provider implementation of best practices in communication and can institute additional educational initiatives and incentives to encourage adoption of these practices. Health plans, health insurance organizations, and Medicare prescription benefits plans will need to develop assessment tools similar to those of other customer service industries but that include the attributes described above. An example of a self-assessment tool recently developed for health insurers is the Health Plan Organizational Assessment of Health Literacy Activities developed by Gazmararian and colleagues for America's Health Insurance Plans (America's Health Insurance Plans, n.d.; Gazmararian et al., 2010). This tool assesses health plans in six areas: printed member information, Web navigation, member services/verbal communication, forms, nurse call lines, and member case/disease management.

4. Commission and Actively Engage a Health literacy Advisory Group That Represents the Target Populations

Too often end users with limited literacy skills are consulted only for the evaluation component of an intervention in order to assess established curricula or else are never consulted at all. As a concrete example of community engagement, health literate organizations can involve health literacy advisory groups in the development and implementation of clear communication strategies and in the formulation of organizational policies around health literacy and clear communication. The advisory group can also participate in needs assessments, review educational materials, test new health IT applications, and be part of the evaluation team assessing the successes of an organization's health literacy programming. Health literate health organizations involve members of lower-literacy populations, adult educators, and experts in health literacy in the development, implementation, and assessment of communication strategies and in ensuring that user-centered design principles are adhered to and that members of the target community are key collaborators in intervention design and implementation. Management teams can commission an advisory group of community literacy experts (including educators and limited-literacy populations) for this purpose. For example, the Department of Health and Human Service's *National Action Plan to Improve Health Literacy* highlights the collaborative efforts of the Iowa Health System and the New Readers of Iowa as an exemplary model for partnering with community-based organizations as a means of enabling community involvement, guidance, and oversight regarding health literacy activities (HHS, 2010). Some advisory groups evolve into ongoing patient learning resource centers or serve as key connectors to community adult literacy programs.

5. Provide the Infrastructure to Avail Frontline Providers, Patients and Families with a Package of Appropriate, High-Quality Educational Supports and Resources

While frontline clinicians can develop the skills and attitudes to be clear and effective communicators and to assess patients' level of comprehension and preparedness, they cannot independently provide the depth, quality, and complexity of communication needed for every patient and every situation, nor can they consistently and reliably carry out the iterative assessments and educational efforts required to maximize patient understanding and skill acquisition over time. Health literate health care organizations recognize that promoting patient comprehension and building patient skills requires high-quality human, technical, and pedagogical resources that are easily accessible across the organization. As such, they provide clinicians and patients access to a functional infrastructure and a package of high-quality educational supports, including written materials, video material, online material, and in-person and group-level education that adheres to clear communication and user-centered design principles. While adjunctive written health information serves as a critical method of reinforcing health knowledge and behaviors introduced during in-person interactions, it can only serve as such if its language, content, and design elements facilitate comprehension. Health literate health care organizations can also establish a formal process of involving the members of the low-literacy community via a health literacy advisory board in planning, developing, and testing written health information to ensure appropriateness. Multiple tools are available to assist health educators and administrators tasked with developing health-related written materials (NCI, 1994). Key components include attention to the use of simple, everyday words; short sentences; appropriate graphics; and well-designed layouts. There should also be a focus on the content of the health material, with an emphasis on "chunking" information into discrete, manageable, content and focusing on actionable health items rather than general information.

Health literate health care organizations make a commitment to providing patients and families with communication and educational support beyond the face-to-face clinician visit to the greatest extent possible. This support can involve visit preparation, post-visit reinforcement, self-management support, decision support, and educational reinforcement during transitions in care. This requires a health literate health care organization to develop a functional educational infrastructure to support providers, patients, and caregivers. Ideally, many educational materials, decision aids, and supports are linked to the organization's electronic health record. While there are many institutions and organizations that produce such material, to our knowledge there is no single clearinghouse that provides an all-encompassing compendium of health literacy–appropriate material. There are, however, publicly available websites for patient education that provide certain materials that may be more comprehensible to the average U.S. patient (e.g., Medline-Plus has an easy-to-read icon for material written at the fifth- through eighth-grade levels and "tutorials" written at the fifth- and sixth-grade levels, and it also has an extensive library of materials in Spanish) (NLM, 2012), and some vendors of patient education materials promote the readability of their products. Self-management support programs have been found to be effective for populations with chronic disease and limited health literacy (Baker et al., 2011a; Rothman et al., 2004; Schillinger et al., 2009). Decision aids that use simplified text and complementary video can improve decisional intent in dementia care planning in populations with limited health literacy (Volandes et al., 2007, 2010), and decisional aids developed through participatory methods can improve decision making in breast cancer care, reducing decisional conflict to a greater degree among those with the least knowledge (Belkora et al., 2011a, 2011b). Finally, the use of virtual patient advocates (embodied conversational agents) as health educators as a complement to in-person discharge education has been shown to reduce rehospitalization, with similar benefits across health literacy levels (Bickmore et al., 2009).

Health literate health care organizations have an instrumental role in influencing the marketplace of patient communication products by demanding rigorous testing with and adaptation for populations with limited health literacy and in supporting the development of national certification standards for print and digital material that is accessible to these populations.

6. Leverage Accessible Health Information Technology (IT) to Embed Health Literacy Practices and Support Providers and Patients

Because effective communication can be time-consuming and because of the high variability in both provider communication skills and patient literacy and learning styles, health IT holds significant promise for enabling patients to provide information and for providing patients with assistance in learning about their conditions and treatments, making decisions, and managing their conditions at home. In addition to enabling forms of communication beyond the written word (visual aids, spoken word), health IT can provide both standardized and tailored information based on patient information or needs and can carry out iterative education to ensure comprehension and mastery, thereby embedding an established health literacy practice. If developed and pretested with populations with limited health literacy, such health IT applications can be highly effective and provide opportunities to deliver education and elicit communication across multiple modalities. Examples include automated telephony for diabetes self-management in the home (Schillinger et al., 2009) and embodied conversational agents for discharge instructions at the bedside (Bickmore et al., 2009). These types of applications can be employed across a range of patient informational and communication needs and strategies, such as pre-visit preparation, after-care summaries, or proactive outreach for health care maintenance, appointment keeping, or medication adherence, among others. AHRQ is currently supporting an effort to develop a set of standards to determine the attributes of electronic health communication resources that make them appropriate for populations with limited health literacy. As described above, health literate health care organizations not only show a willingness to employ such innovations, but they also participate in the innovation process by adapting them to the needs of patients with limited health literacy or requiring that vendors of such applications have demonstrated their effectiveness with these populations before purchasing them.

7. Provide Patient Training and Assistance Around Personal Health Records and Health IT Tools

eHealth literacy refers to the "ability to seek, find, understand, and appraise information from electronic sources and apply this knowledge to addressing or solving a health problem" (Norman and Skinner, 2006). Patients with limited health literacy often have low eHealth literacy. One specific form of interactive health IT, personal electronic health records (pEHRs), gives patients the ability to store and access personal health information, interact with their providers, and receive electronic educational resources. While these technological advances can improve access to health information and advance self-management in some cases, their introduction may widen communication disparities between those patients with adequate health literacy skills and those without. A recent study found that having limited literacy skills was independently associated with significantly lower rates of using a personal health record to make appointments, review medication regimens, refill medications, check laboratory results, or e-mail one's provider, even among those with Internet access (Sarkar et al., 2010a).

Health literate health care organizations take steps to ensure that patients with low health and eHealth literacy are able to benefit from technological advances. Health literate health care organizations advocate that IT firms developing pEHR implement best practices in health IT, including simple home page design with minimal text per screen, use of HTML for websites, a consistent and simple navigation approach, simplified search tools, a minimized need for scrolling, the availability of printer-friendly options, and easy-to-find contact information (Eichner and Dullabh, 2007). Health literate health care organizations should solicit input from the target community on the development and selection of pEHR systems. A detailed checklist has been developed by the National Resource Center for Health IT and AHRQ (Eichner and Dullabh, 2007); health literate health care organizations adhere to these recommendations when developing their own applications and when purchasing products from vendors. Health literate health care organizations implement educational initiatives so that end users can be oriented, assisted, trained, and motivated in pEHR use to the greatest extent possible. Finally, because the diffusion of digital innovations will be slower among populations with limited health literacy, health literate health care organizations do not supplant human connection with digital options; information and education available on pEHR should also be accessible through interpersonal means.

8. Foster an Augmented and Prepared Workforce to Promote Health Literacy

The current structure of the U.S. health care system places emphasis of communication and education on the physician provider. Patients with limited health literacy report suboptimal verbal communication with their physicians (HRSA, n.d.; Schillinger et al., 2004). As care delivery shifts toward the patient-centered medical home model and accountable care organizations, health literate health care organizations should diversify their provider workforce and expand job descriptions in line with the variety of educational roles that nonphysician members of the health care team will serve in patient-centered health homes. Priority should be placed on hiring and integrating health educators, health coaches, social workers, patient navigators, nurses, medical assistants, and even peers into health management and health education roles. Health literate health care organizations should also ensure that members of the health care team reflect the socio-demographic profiles of the patient populations served as another means to improve trust and communication. Health literate organizations should also develop "expert educators" with cross-cutting educational skills who can teach others how to teach, can teach about specific medical conditions, can help evaluate the educational and communication needs of patients to refine or identify appropriate new curricula, and can serve as organizational contacts to identify electronic educational resources. These approaches to redesigning the workforce, however logical, will require evaluation to demonstrate a return on investment, as their effectiveness in reducing health literacy–related disparities has not been well studied (Sheridan et al., 2011).

A health literate health care organization provides health literacy and health communication training for all members of the integrated health team: receptionists, team members tasked with helping patients enroll in insurance benefits or receive social services, case managers, and all medical providers. The goal of this training is to provide all members of the team with basic competencies in clear communication and the ability to recognize when patients have communication barriers for which clear communication is insufficient and thus need more intensive communication support. Through widespread training, health literate organizations can establish a culture in which all members of the health care team work with the unified goal of promoting open communication with patients. Health care team members specifically tasked with health education roles should receive more detailed training in educational techniques that help patients achieve mastery over health care material. A number of comprehensive and well designed health literacy educational modules are available online (AMA, 2007b; DeWalt et al., 2010; HRSA, n.d.; New York New Jersey Public Health Training Center, 2011).

Health literacy experts have identified a number of best practices in communication that all members of the health care team can employ when interacting with patients. These include the following:

- Assessing patient comprehension of pre-specified knowledge domains and ability to demonstrate specific skills
- Avoiding medical jargon and using plain, everyday ("living room") language in conversation
- Limiting the amount of information introduced in each conversation
- Prioritizing learning goals to two to three concepts per visit
- Actively eliciting patient's symptoms and concerns
- Using the "teach back," "teach to goal," and "show me" methods (Schillinger et al., 2003) to ensure patient comprehension and skills. This has been identified as a top safety practice by the National Quality Forum (National Quality Forum, 2005, 2010).
- Encouraging the asking of questions
- Focusing on information that is actionable

9. Distribute Resources to Better Meet the Needs of the Populations Served

The inverse care hypothesis, a concept that has been applied to explain health care disparities, states that the availability and quality of health care tends to vary inversely with the needs of the population (Schillinger, 2007). Health literate health care organizations, however, recognize that the distribution of the health literacy workforce across the organization should be commensurate with the local needs of the populations served. As such, health literate health care organizations reallocate existing resources or allocate additional resources to underperforming regions or sites so that underperformance attributable to a disproportionate concentration of patients with limited health literacy can be improved upon.

This approach to the allocation of resources extends to educational and communication initiatives. Health literate health care organizations provide an intensity and interactivity of communication that is proportional to the communication needs of the patients it is targeting. Curricular approaches, such as the "teach-to-goal" method described below (Baker et al., 2011b), is an example of distributing more educational resources (time and effort) to those who need more. Other strategies, such as automated telephonic proactive outreach, can deliver more education and interaction between visits for those with greater communication needs, thereby helping patients achieve behavioral goals (Schillinger et al., 2008).

10. Employ a Higher Standard to Ensure Understanding of High-Risk Decisions and High-Risk Transitions

While promoting patient understanding through well-written health information, understandable verbal communication, and visual aids is a core value of health literate health care organizations, there are high-risk decisions in health care and important transitions that demand a heightened level of assurance that patients (or their surrogates, if the patient is not competent) fully understand. Health literate health care organizations often have identified which common decisions merit this degree of scrutiny and have standards and processes in place to ensure that comprehension has been accomplished, often by embedding health literacy practices, such as exposure to a standardized and well-designed teaching tool combined with successful demonstration (and documentation) of comprehension of key learning objectives using the teach-back method. Examples of high-risk circumstances include, but are not limited to, informed consent for surgery; administration of medications with serious complications or "black box" warnings, such as chemotherapy drugs, anticoagulants, immunosuppressive agents, or thrombolytic agents; and transitions in care, such as a discharge from the hospital. Hospital discharge processes can be improved by asking patients to "explain in your own words" the reason they were in the hospital and what they need to do to take care of themselves when they return home. Prior to surgery patients can be asked to "explain in your own words" the name of the surgery; the reason that it is being done; and the hoped-for benefits, likelihood of success, and possible risks. These responses offer an opportunity for continued dialogue and education around a critical moment. Patients' responses can also be included in the consent and discharge paperwork as documentation of clear communication and comprehension. Efforts by the Iowa Health System that are highlighted in the AMA manual *Health Literacy and Patient Safety: Help Patients Understand* provide an example of such a modified consent form (AMA, 2007b).

11. Prioritize Medication Safety and Medication Communication

A host of studies have shown that patients with low health literacy are more likely to misunderstand prescription drug labels (e.g., Wolf et al., 2007); that they have difficulty understanding drug warnings (Davis et al., 2006), using nonstandardized dosing instruments (Yin et al., 2007), have difficulty effectively consolidating medication regimens if dosing instructions are variable ("every 12 hours" versus "twice a day") (Sarkar et al., 2010b; Wolf et al., 2011a), and err in taking medication in the post-discharge context (unintentional non-adherence) (Lindquist et al., 2011) or in the diabetes context (severe hypoglycemia) (Sarkar et al., 2010b); and that they are less able to identify their medications (Kripalani et al., 2006). Additional factors, such as poor understanding regarding medication costs, changing formularies, nonstandard prescribing factors, confusion regarding generic and brand name labeling, and changing medication colors and shapes, make safe medication management even more difficult.

A health literate health care organization prioritizes medication safety by implementing systems and interventions that advance medication safety and self-management. In-person medication reconciliation, such as "brown-bag medication reviews," provides an opportunity for patients to bring in all of their medications, including over-the-counter medications, and review how and why they take each of their medications. It is an opportunity for providers—including, but not limited to, pharmacists—to identify medication errors, such as duplicate medications; to reduce medication burden in the case of poly-pharmacy; and to identify patients who need extra time for medication teaching. Any provider trained with "show me" skills can help implement brown-bag reviews. The goals are not only to ensure that the regimen is accurate, but also to reinforce patients' ability to answer the questions. How do I take my medicine, what is it for, and why is it important for me to take it? Health literate health care organizations recognize that medication reviews, if well done, are time-consuming and require incentivizing providers with the time and reimbursement to carry them out.

Health literate health care organizations establish internal guidelines on prescribing, including using standardized times and the consistent use of plain language, without abbreviations, in all medication prescriptions. Wolf and colleagues (2011b) have published promising work showing that standardized labels, with prescribing instructions centered around four standard time periods and universal language standards, can improve low-literacy patients' ability to dose medications correctly and can improve their ability to consolidate complex regimens into more feasible daily schedules. Further advances in this field may be supported by changes in the national guidelines for prescription standards. Because research suggests that embedding visual aids (pill images) into medication counseling and labeling can reduce medication-taking errors (Machtinger et al., 2007), health literate health care organizations employ such visual aids to enhance safety.

Finally, recognizing that the complexities related to health insurance benefits and medication cost coverage and co-payments affect most profoundly those with limited health literacy. Health literate health care organizations provide prescribing providers with up-to-date information regarding which medications are covered by a patient's health insurance so as to reduce the likelihood that patients will have to unnecessarily navigate prior-authorization procedures. These organizations also provide staff and resources to patients to help them make decisions regarding medication options and drug plan options.

12. Make Health Plan and Health Insurance Products More Transparent and Comprehensible

As the health care industry becomes even more multi-sectoral, patients and their families are being asked to navigate choices and overcome barriers related to health insurance, health providers, and health services and to help in making a greater number of decisions regarding their care that go beyond traditional clinical decision making. As the Patient Protection and Affordable Care Act (ACA) is put into effect, many Americans—a large portion of whom will have limited health literacy—will need to make decisions about health coverage plans. Decision making in the face of medical, financial, and administrative complexity will be overwhelming and burdensome for many. Ensuring that patients with limited health literacy successfully enroll is fundamental to the success of health care reform. Health literate health care organizations, including insurance plans, insurance exchanges, and pharmacy benefits management companies, provide information about benefits packages that is readily available to patients and their families, ensure that this information is understandable, and establish straightforward methods for patients and families to access in-person support for additional assistance.

Recently proposed regulations regarding the Health Insurance Exchange will assist patients in deciding between health insurance plans. The regulation requires that patients have access to an easy-to-understand summary of benefits and coverage and to a glossary of terms related to health insurance coverage (HHS, 2011; U.S. Department of Labor, 2011).

The California Medicaid program (Medi-Cal) recently partnered with the University of California–Berkeley School of Public Health to help seniors and people with disabilities understand their Medi-Cal health care choices, using participatory design to create a guidebook in English, Spanish, and Chinese that explains enrollment options and benefits. An evaluation showed that the guidebook increased understanding of enrollment options and the capacity to make choices (Neuhauser et al., 2009).

13. Make Systems More Navigable and Support Patients and Families in Navigating the Health Care System

Navigation within the health care system involves interacting with the built environment and finding one's way between locations. In addition, it requires an ability to accomplish the myriad tasks needed to manage health within an increasingly complicated and fragmented medical system. It involves scheduling specialist appointments, enrolling for insurance services, understanding one's health care benefits, dealing with pharmacy benefits management companies, finding locations for diagnostic studies, and connecting with community agencies. Health literate health care organizations work at establishing a shame-free environment so that patients and their families will be comfortable asking for help when needed. Employing clear signage and designing patient-friendly office procedures, including establishing a welcoming environment; offering assistance with all literacy-related tasks, such as reading and completing forms; and assisting patients with scheduling and finding referral and diagnostic test locations can help overcome these challenges.

Examples of design interventions that have made systems more navigable, especially for populations with limited health literacy, include electronic referrals to specialists (Kim-Hwang et al., 2010), which minimize the burden on patients to aggregate and master complex health information related to their consultations. Medical homes, with their promise of "one-stop-shopping," can also simplify service delivery. The One-e-App program, an innovative web-based system, provides an efficient one-stop approach to enrollment in a range of public and private health, social service, and other support programs. One-e-App streamlines the application process through one electronic application that collects and stores information, screens and delivers data electronically, and helps families connect to needed services (California HealthCare Foundation, 2012).

Organization leadership can also enlist a team to perform an environmental assessment as a means of identifying areas in the built environment that may represent literacy barriers, such as poor or absent signage; absence of navigational guides, including maps; inconsistent labeling of locations and services; and lack of present and available personnel who can provide assistance (Rudd and Anderson, 2006; Sarkar et al., 2010a). These types of assessments are not just the responsibility of traditional health care delivery units (e.g., hospital or ambulatory clinic) but also of organizations in the health insurance industry, whose processes for enrollment, billing, prior authorization, and claims are notoriously difficult to navigate, often redundant, and generally confusing.

14. Recognize Social Needs as Medical Concerns and Connect People to Community Resources

Individuals with limited health literacy are often subject to other social vulnerabilities. These social needs, including housing instability, food insecurity, lack of transportation, unemployment, social isolation, legal concerns, and interpersonal violence, often have direct medical consequences and affect patients' ability to effectively engage in self-management. However, members of the health team often miss the opportunity to assess patients for these conditions (Fleegler et al., 2007). Even when providers do identify social needs, health systems may not have the infrastructure and manpower to connect patients to needed social services.

There are some examples of efforts by health care organizations to partner with community resources. The Health Leads program (Health Leads, 2011; Robert Wood Johnson Foundation, 2011), a volunteer-driven program based in outpatient clinics, allows medical providers to "prescribe" social service needs such as food, housing, and job training. The prescription is then "filled" by one of the college volunteers who work with patients to connect them with needed social services and who can continue to follow up in the event that there is additional need. The Robert Wood Johnson Foundation and AHRQ's collaborative Prescription for Health initiative funded community-based projects to explore how primary care practices can make linkages with community resources to promote healthy behavior. While many of these projects were successful, an overall analysis of these programs suggests that sustaining linkages required continued communications between the health care system and the community resources and argues for a system in which clinical services and community services are integrated (Etz et al., 2008; Woolf et al., 2005). At a minimum health systems can develop a clearinghouse of local resources, identify members of the health care team to become champions in connecting with resources, and partner with case managers or social workers to assist with linking patients to resources.

Ultimately, unaddressed "non-health" social needs of patients will prevent patients from fully benefiting from the health care system and partnering in care. A health literate organization views linking patients with social resources as a fundamental part of providing medical care and ensures that there are systems in place to ensure that these connections are made.

15. Create a Climate in Which Asking Questions Is Encouraged and Expected

Patients with limited health literacy have been found to be less likely to ask questions of their providers or to have interactive communication in a visit. They may not disclose their challenges with reading and comprehension due to shame (Parikh et al., 1996). Interventions to "activate" patients to be more involved and to advocate for themselves hold promise as a means to increase the asking of questions and interactivity. Health literate health care organizations encourage and expect patients to be asking questions of their health care teams. The National Safety Foundation's Ask Me 3 campaign attempts to facilitate communication between patients and providers by encouraging patients to ask the following questions:

1. What is my main problem?
2. What do I need to do?
3. Why is it important for me to do this? (National Patient Safety Foundation, n.d.)

Orienting providers to these questions, displaying posters, and distributing brochures encouraging the use of the Ask Me 3 questions may be an effective step in empowering patients to ask more questions, especially when it is linked with clinician training in health literacy, including the importance of minimizing patient shame (Mika et al., 2007). Additional resources, such as the AHRQ's "Questions are the Answers" website (AHRQ, n.d.) can help patients formulate a list of questions to remember to ask their providers during a medical visit. Both of these initiatives can be strengthened by having allied members of the health care team encourage and remind patients to think of questions while preparing for their visits and to focus learning around these questions between visits.

16. Develop and Implement Curricula to Develop Mastery of a Threshold-Level Set of Knowledge and Skills

In order to improve skill building and to help patients reach behavioral goals as well as to track patient progress over time and across settings, health literate health care organizations develop curricular programs that acknowledge and are designed around the learning constraints related to patients' working memory (generally a fixed capacity) and cognitive load (the learning demands, based on the complexities and quantity of the material). Baker and colleagues (2011b) describe six principles in helping patients achieve their learning goals:

1. Define a limited set of critical learning goals and eliminate all other information that does not directly support the learning goals.
2. Present information in discrete, predetermined "chunks."
3. Determine the optimal order for teaching the topics.
4. Develop plain-language text to explain essential concepts for each goal, and employ appropriate graphics to increase comprehension and recall.
5. Confirm understanding after each unit, perform tailored instruction until mastery is attained, and review previously learned concepts until stable mastery is achieved.
6. Link all instruction to a specific attitude, skill, or behavioral goal.

These principles can be integrated into health-education initiatives in multiple health care settings being executed by a variety of providers, including physicians, nutritionists, pharmacists, health-at-home providers, and health educators. Having agreement on a shared curriculum can facilitate continued, consistent, and complementary education in different settings and across time to reinforce and build skills to approach mastery.

17. Continually Assess and Track Patient Comprehension, Skills, and Ability to Problem-Solve Around Health Conditions

While health literate health care organizations create "shame-free" environments where the asking of questions by patients is encouraged and expected, these organizations also build in procedures and systems to periodically assess and document patient comprehension and basic problem-solving skills across a range of common conditions that rely on self-management. Exemplar conditions include congestive heart failure, diabetes, asthma/chronic obstructive pulmonary disease, and anticoagulant care. Examples of skills and abilities important when dealing with heart failure include knowing one's target weight, knowing what is involved in a daily self-check (e.g., leg swelling, weight change, changes in patterns of shortness of breath, and lightheadedness or dizziness), and knowing how to self-titrate one's diuretic pill and when to call the medical home to prevent deterioration (Baker at al., 2011b; DeWalt et al., 2009). Examples pertaining to anticoagulant care for stroke prevention include knowing the signs and symptoms of stroke, knowing the recommended frequencies of blood testing and their meanings, accurately reporting one's anticoagulant regimen, being aware that the anticoagulant medications interact with many others medications and therefore require vigilance, and recognizing the clinical relevance of bleeding (Fang et al., 2006). Such assessments can identify individuals at risk for poor comprehension, target immediate educational efforts, and provide an indication for additional educational supports so that improvements or even mastery can be achieved over time. These assessments can also serve as valuable and dynamic information to share with the broader health care team working to improve a patient's health literacy so that educational efforts reinforce, rather than compete with, each other and so that progress can be tracked. These efforts may also identify individuals with heretofore unrecognized and common learning barriers beyond limited literacy skills, such as cognitive impairment, learning disabilities, and hearing or visual impairment.

18. Recognize and Accommodate Additional Barriers to Communication

Limited health literacy is one of a number of common communication challenges patients face. Limited English proficiency, cognitive decline, hearing and visual impairment, learning disabilities, and mental health problems all may create barriers to clear communication. Many of these communication barriers travel together. When these challenges overlap, such barriers tend to compound or even overwhelm literacy-related obstacles (Sudore et al., 2009). A health literate health care organization prioritizes providing culturally and linguistically competent care and seeks to implement guidelines and recommendations for culturally and linguistically appropriate services (HHS, 2001). Health literate organizations recruit and cultivate a culturally and linguistically diverse staff and provide training in best practices working with medical interpreters for all members of the health care team. These organizations also have resources and procedures in place to identify and remediate hearing loss and visual impairment as well as to identify cognitive impairment that would require case management or engagement of surrogates and family caregivers.

CONCLUSION

Despite a growing understanding that health literacy challenges represent a mismatch between patients' health literacy skills and the literacy demands of the greater health care system, until recently the majority of health literacy efforts have focused on interventions directed to the patient. The opportunities for systems redesign surrounding the implementation of the Patient Protection and Affordable Care Act, including health insurance exchanges and Medicaid expansion, the advanced medical home, accountable care organizations, and health IT expansion, provide momentum for organizations to integrate principles of health literacy into organizational objectives, infrastructure, policies and practices, workforce development, and communication strategies. In this paper, we introduce a set of attributes, goals, and foci for institutional investment that health literate health care organizations can embrace to begin to address the system-level factors that can prevent patients and families from fully benefiting from the health care system. This list of attributes and goals, which is by no means exhaustive, provides a roadmap for organizational change and relates most clearly to organizations that provide direct care to patients. However, a majority of the goals and attributes are also relevant to the broader range of organizations, stakeholders, and institutions that comprise the modern health care system. We see this paper less as the definitive response to the challenge of defining a "health literate health care organization" and more as an attempt to advance an optimistic vision of how organizations should evolve to be more responsive to the needs of populations with limited health literacy in tangible ways, thereby improving care for all.

REFERENCES

AHRQ (Agency for Healthcare Research). n.d. *Questions Are the Answer*. http://www.ahrq.gov/questions/ (accessed March 21, 2012).

Allen, K., J. Zoellner, M. Motley, and P. A. Estabrooks. 2011. Understanding the internal and external validity of health literacy interventions: A systematic literature review using the RE-AIM framework. *Journal of Health Communication* 16(Suppl 3):55–72.

AMA (American Medical Association). 2007a. *Health Literacy and Patient Safety: Help Patients Understand (Manual for Clinicians)*. http://www.ama-assn.org/ama1/pub/upload/mm/367/healthlitclinicians.pdf (accessed March 21, 2012).

AMA. 2007b. *Health Literacy and Patient Safety: Help Patients Understand*. http://www.ama-assn.org/ama/pub/about-ama/ama-foundation/our-programs/public-health/health-literacy-program/health-literacy-kit.

America's Health Insurance Plans. n.d. *Health Plan Organizational Assessment of Health Literacy Activities, Resource List—Health Plan Organizational Assessment of Health Literacy Activities, and Suggestions for Areas of Improvement*. http://www.ahip.org/content/default.aspx?docid=29467.

Baker, D. W., R. M. Parker, M. V. Williams, W. S. Clark, and J. Nurss. 1997. The relationship of patient reading ability to self-reported health and use of health services. *American Journal of Public Health* 87(6):1027–1030.

Baker, D. W., J. A. Gazmararian, M. V. Williams, T. Scott, R. M. Parker, D. Green, J. Ren, and J. Peel. 2002. Functional health literacy and the risk of hospital admission among Medicare managed care enrollees. *American Journal of Public Health* 92(8):1278–1283.

Baker, D. W., D. A. Dewalt, D. Schillinger, V. Hawk, B. Ruo, K. Bibbins-Domingo, M. Weinberger, A. Macabasco-O'Connell, K. L. Grady, G. M. Holmes, B. Erman, K. A. Broucksou, and M. Pignone. 2011a. The effect of progressive, reinforcing telephone education and counseling versus brief educational intervention on knowledge, self-care behaviors and heart failure symptoms. *Journal of Cardiac Failure* 17(10):789–796.

Baker, D. W., D. A. Dewalt, D. Schillinger, V. Hawk, B. Ruo, K. Bibbins-Domingo, M. Weinberger, A. Macabasco-O'Connell, and M. Pignone. 2011b. "Teach to goal": Theory and design principles of an intervention to improve heart failure self-management skills of patients with low health literacy. *Journal of Health Communication* 16(Suppl 3):73–88.

Belkora, J. K., A. Teng, S. Volz, M. K. Loth, and L. J. Esserman. 2011a. Expanding the reach of decision and communication aids in a breast care center: A quality improvement study. *Patient Education and Counseling* 83(2):234–239.

Belkora, J. K., S. Volz, A. E. Teng, D. H. Moore, M. K. Loth, and K. R. Sepucha. 2011b. Impact of decision aids in a sustained implementation at a breast care center. *Patient Education and Counseling* 86(2):195–204.

Bickmore, T. W., L. M. Pfeifer, and M. K. Paasche-Orlow. 2009. Using computer agents to explain medical documents to patients with low health literacy. *Patient Education and Counseling* 75(3):315–320.

California HealthCare Foundation. 2012. *One-e-App: One-Stop Access to Health and Social Service Programs*. http://www.chcf.org/projects/2007/oneeapp-onestop-access-to-health-care (accessed March 21, 2012).

Cavanaugh, K., M. M. Huizinga, K. A. Wallston, T. Gebretsadik, A. Shintani, D. Davis, R. P. Gregory, L. Fuchs, R. Malone, A. Cherrington, M. Pignone, D. A. DeWalt, T. A. Elasy, and R. L. Rothman. 2008. Association of numeracy and diabetes control. *Annals of Internal Medicine* 148(10):737–746.

Davis, T. C., M. S. Wolf, P. F. Bass, 3rd, M. Middlebrooks, E. Kennen, D. W. Baker, C. L. Bennett, R. Durazo-Arvizu, A. Bocchini, S. Savory, and R. M. Parker. 2006. Low literacy impairs comprehension of prescription drug warning labels. *Journal of General Internal Medicine* 21(8):847–851.

DeWalt, D. A., K. A. Broucksou, V. Hawk, D. W. Baker, D. Schillinger, B. Ruo, K. Bibbins-Domingo, M. Holmes, M. Weinberger, A. Macabasco-O'Connell, and M. Pignone. 2009. Comparison of a one-time educational intervention to a teach-to-goal educational intervention for self-management of heart failure: Design of a randomized controlled trial. *BMC Health Services Research* 9:99. http://www.ncbi.nlm.nih.gov/pmc/articles/PMC2702288/?tool=pubmed (accessed March 21, 2012).

DeWalt, D. A., L. F. Callahan, V. H. Hawk, K. A. Broucksou, A. Hink, R. Rudd, and C. Brach. 2010. *Health Literacy Universal Precautions Toolkit. Prepared for Agency for Healthcare Research and Quality*. http://www.ahrq.gov/qual/literacy/healthliteracytoolkit.pdf (accessed March 21, 2012).

Eichner, J, and P. Dullabh. 2007. *Accessible Health Information Technology (Health IT) for Populations with Limited Literacy: A Guide for Developers and Purchasers of Health IT*. Rockville, MD: Agency for Healthcare Research and Quality.

Etz, R. S., D. J. Cohen, S. H. Woolf, J. Summers Holtrop, K. E. Donahue, N. F. Isaacson, K. C. Stange, R. L. Ferrer, and A. L. Olson. 2008. Bridging primary care practices and communities to promote healthy behaviors. *American Journal of Preventive Medicine* 35(5 Suppl):S390–S397.

Fang, M. C., E. L. Machtinger, F. Wang, and D. Schillinger. 2006. Health literacy and anticoagulation-related outcomes among patients taking warfarin. *Journal of General Internal Medicine* 21(8):841–846.

Fleegler, E. W., T. A. Lieu, P. H. Wise, and S. Muret-Wagstaff. 2007. Families' health-related social problems and missed referral opportunities. *Pediatrics* 119(6):e1332–e1341.

Gazmararian, J. A., K. Beditz, S. Pisano, and R. Carreon. 2010. The development of a health literacy assessment tool for health plans. *Journal of Health Communication* 15(Suppl 2):93–101.

Hardie, N. A., K. Kyanko, S. Busch, A. T. Losasso, and R. A. Levin. 2011. Health literacy and health care spending and utilization in a consumer-driven health plan. *Journal of Health Communication* 16(Suppl 3):308–321.

Health Leads. 2011. *A New Vision for Healthcare in America*. http://www.healthleadsusa.org/ (accessed March 21, 2012).

HHS (U.S. Department of Health and Human Services). 2001. *National Standards for Culturally and Linguistically Appropriate Services in Health Care*. Washington, DC: U.S. Department of Health and Human Services.

HHS. 2010. *National Action Plan to Improve Health Literacy*. Washington, DC: U.S. Department of Health and Human Services. http://www.health.gov/communication/HLActionPlan/ (accessed March 21, 2012).

HHS. 2011. *Providing Clear and Consistent Information to Consumers about Their Health Insurance Coverage*. http://www.healthcare.gov/news/factsheets/2011/08/labels08172011a.html (accessed March 12, 2012).

HRSA (Health Resources and Services Administration). n.d. *Unified Health Communication (UHC): Addressing Health Literacy, Cultural Competency, and Limited English Proficiency*. http://www.hrsa.gov/publichealth/healthliteracy/index.html (accessed March 21, 2012).

IOM (Institute of Medicine). 2004. Health Literacy: A Prescription to End Confusion. Edited by L. Nielsen-Bohlman, A. Panzer, and D. A. Kindig. Washington, DC: The National Academies Press.

Jacobson, K. L., J. A. Gazmararian, S. Kripalani, K. J. McMorris, S. C. Blake, and C. Brach. 2007. *Is Our Pharmacy Meeting Patients' Needs? A Pharmacy Health Literacy Assessment Tool User's Guide*. Rockville, MD: Agency for Healthcare Research and Quality.

Joint Commission. 2007. *What Did the Doctor Say? Improving Health Literacy to Protect Patient Safety*. http://www.jointcommission.org/What_Did_the_Doctor_Say/ (accessed March 21, 2012).

Kim-Hwang, J. E., A. H. Chen, D. S. Bell, D. Guzman, H. F. Yee, Jr., and M. B. Kushel. 2010. Evaluating electronic referrals for specialty care at a public hospital. *Journal of General Internal Medicine* 25(10):1123–1128.

Kripalani, S., L. E. Henderson, E. Y. Chiu, R. Robertson, P. Kolm, and T. A. Jacobson. 2006. Predictors of medication self-management skill in a low-literacy population. *Journal of General Internal Medicine* 21(8):852–856.

Lindquist, L. A., L. Go, J. Fleisher, N. Jain, E. Friesema, and D. W. Baker. 2011. Relationship of health literacy to intentional and unintentional non-adherence of hospital discharge medications. *Journal of General Internal Medicine* 27(2):173–178.

Machtinger, E. L., F. Wang, L.-L. Chen, M. Rodriguez, S. Wu, and D. Schillinger. 2007. A visual medication schedule to improve anticoagulation control: A randomized, controlled trial. *Joint Commission Journal on Quality and Patient Safety/Joint Commission Resources* 33(10):625–635.

Martin, L. T., and R. M. Parker. 2011. Insurance expansion and health literacy. *JAMA* 306(8):874–875.

Mika, V. S., P. R. Wood, B. D. Weiss, and L. Treviño. 2007. Ask Me 3: Improving communication in a Hispanic pediatric outpatient practice. *American Journal of Health Behavior* 31(Suppl 1):S115–S121.

National Center for Education Statistics. 2006. *The Health Literacy of America's Adults: Results From the 2003 National Assessment of Adult Literacy*. Washington, DC: U.S. Department of Education.

National Patient Safety Foundation. n.d. *Ask Me 3*. Available from http://www.npsf.org/askme3/ (accessed March 21, 2012).

National Quality Forum. 2005. *Improving Patient Safety Through Informed Consent for Patients with Limited Health Literacy*. Washington, DC: National Quality Forum.

National Quality Forum. 2009 (March). *Health Literacy: A Linchpin in Achieving National Goals for Health and Healthcare*. Washington, DC: National Quality Forum.

National Quality Forum. 2010. *Safe Practices for Better Healthcare—2010 Update*. Washington DC: National Quality Forum.

NCI (National Cancer Institute). 1994. *Clear & Simple: Developing Effective Print Materials for Low-Literate Readers*. Bethesda, MD: National Cancer Institute.

Neuhauser, L., B. Rothschild, C. Graham, S. L. Ivey, and S. Konishi. 2009. Participatory design of mass health communication in three languages for seniors and people with disabilities on Medicaid. *American Journal of Public Health* 99(12):2188–2195.

New York New Jersey Public Health Training Center. 2011. *Health Literacy & Public Health: Strategies for Addressing Low Health Literacy*. http://www.nynj-phtc.org/pages/catalog/phlit02/ (accessed March 21, 2012).

NLM (National Library of Medicine). 2012. *Easy-to-Read Health Materials*. http://www.nlm.nih.gov/medlineplus/all_easytoread.html (accessed March 21, 2012).

Norman, C. D., and H. A. Skinner. 2006. eHEALS: The eHealth Literacy Scale. *Journal of Medical Internet Research* 8(4):e27–e27.

Parikh, N. S., R. M. Parker, J. R. Nurss, D. W. Baker, and M. V. Williams. 1996. Shame and health literacy: The unspoken connection. *Patient Education and Counseling* 27(1):33–39.

Robert Wood Johnson Foundation. 2011. *An Innovative Prescription for Better Health*. http://www.rwjf.org/vulnerablepopulations/product.jsp?id=72319 (accessed March 21, 2012).

Rothman, R. L., D. A. DeWalt, R. Malone, B. Bryant, A. Shintani, B. Crigler, M. Weinberger, and M. Pignone. 2004. Influence of patient literacy on the effectiveness of a primary care-based diabetes disease management program. *JAMA* 292(14):1711–1716.

Rudd, R., and J. Anderson. 2006. *The Health Literacy Environment of Hospitals and Health Centers. National Center for the Study of Adult Learning and Literacy 2006*. http://www.hsph.harvard.edu/healthliteracy/files/healthliteracyenvironment.pdf (accessed March 21, 2012)

Sarkar, U., J. D. Piette, R. Gonzales, D. Lessler, L. D. Chew, B. Reilly, J. Johnson, M. Brunt, J. Huang, M. Regenstein, and D. Schillinger. 2008. Preferences for self-management support: Findings from a survey of diabetes patients in safety-net health systems. *Patient Education and Counseling* 70(1):102–110.

Sarkar, U., A. J. Karter, J. Y. Liu, N. E. Adler, R. Nguyen, A. Lopez, and D. Schillinger. 2010a. The literacy divide: Health literacy and the use of an Internet-based patient portal in an integrated health system-results from The Diabetes Study of Northern California (DISTANCE). *Journal of Health Communication* 15(Suppl 2):183–196.

Sarkar, U., A. J. Karter, J. Y. Liu, H. H. Moffet, N. E. Adler, and D. Schillinger. 2010b. Hypoglycemia is more common among type 2 diabetes patients with limited health literacy: The Diabetes Study of Northern California (DISTANCE). *Journal of General Internal Medicine* 25(9):962–968.

Sarkar, U., D. Schillinger, K. Bibbins–Domingo, A. Nápoles, L. Karliner, and E. J. Pérez-Stable. 2011. Patient-physicians' information exchange in outpatient cardiac care: Time for a heart to heart? *Patient Education and Counseling* 85(2):173–179.

Schillinger, D. 2007. Literacy and health communication: Reversing the "inverse care law." *The American Journal of Bioethics* 7(11):15–18; discussion W1–W2.

Schillinger, D., K. Grumbach, J. Piette, F. Wang, D. Osmond, C. Daher, J. Palacios, G. D. Sullivan, and A. B. Bindman. 2002. Association of health literacy with diabetes outcomes. *JAMA* 288(4):475–482.

Schillinger, D., J. Piette, K. Grumbach, F. Wang, C. Wilson, C. Daher, K. Leong-Grotz, C. Castro, and A. B. Bindman. 2003. Closing the loop: Physician communication with diabetic patients who have low health literacy. *Archives of Internal Medicine* 163(1):83–90.

Schillinger, D., A. Bindman, F. Wang, A. Stewart, and J. Piette. 2004. Functional health literacy and the quality of physician-patient communication among diabetes patients. *Patient Education and Counseling* 52(3):315–323.

Schillinger, D., E. L. Machtinger, F. Wang, L. L. Chen, K. Win, J. Palacios, M. Rodriguez, and A. Bindman. 2005. Language, literacy, and communication regarding medication in an anticoagulation clinic: Are pictures better than words? In K. Henriksen, J. B. Battles, E. S. Marks, and D. I. Lewin, eds. *Advances in Patient Safety: From Research to Implementation, Vol. 2: Concepts and Methodology* (pp. 199–212). Rockville, MD: Agency for Healthcare Research and Quality.

Schillinger, D., H. Hammer, F. Wang, J. Palacios, I. McLean, A. Tang, S. Youmans, and M. Handley. 2008. Seeing in 3-D: Examining the reach of diabetes self-management support strategies in a public health care system. *Health Education & Behavior* 35(5):664–682.

Schillinger, D., M. Handley, F. Wang, and H. Hammer. 2009. Effects of self-management support on structure, process, and outcomes among vulnerable patients with diabetes: A three-arm practical clinical trial. *Diabetes Care* 32(4):559–566.

Sheridan, S. L., D. J. Halpern, A. J. Viera, N. D. Berkman, K. E. Donahue, and K. Crotty. 2011. Interventions for individuals with low health literacy: A systematic review. *Journal of Health Communication* 16(Suppl 3):30–54.

Sommers, B. D., and A. M. Epstein. 2010. Medicaid expansion—the soft underbelly of health care reform? *New England Journal of Medicine* 363(22):2085–2087.

Sudore, R. L., K. Yaffe, S. Satterfield, T. B. Harris, K. M. Mehta, E. M. Simonsick, A. B. Newman, C. Rosano, R. Rooks, S. M. Rubin, H. N. Ayonayon, and D. Schillinger. 2006. Limited literacy and mortality in the elderly: The health, aging, and body composition study. *Journal of General Internal Medicine* 21(8):806–812.

Sudore, R. L., C. S. Landefeld, E. J. Perez-Stable, K. Bibbins-Domingo, B. A. Williams, and D. Schillinger. 2009. Unraveling the relationship between literacy, language proficiency, and patient–physician communication. *Patient Education and Counseling* 75(3):398–402.

U.S. Department of Labor. 2011. *New Affordable Care Act Proposal to Help Consumers Better Understand and Compare Benefits and Coverage*. http://www.dol.gov/opa/media/press/ebsa/EBSA20111232.htm (accessed March 21, 2012).

U.S. Surgeon General. 2006. Paper read at the Surgeon General's Workshop on Improving Health Literacy, September 7, at National Institutes of Health, Bethesda, MD.

Vernon, J., A. Trujillo, S. Rosenbaum, and B. DeBuono. 2007. *Low Health Literacy: Implications for National Health Policy*. National Patient Safety Foundation. http://www.gwumc.edu/sphhs/departments/healthpolicy/CHPR/downloads/LowHealthLiteracyReport10_4_07.pdf (accessed March 21, 2012).

Volandes, A. E., L. S. Lehmann, E. F. Cook, S. Shaykevich, E. D. Abbo, and M. R. Gillick. 2007. Using video images of dementia in advance care planning. *Archives of Internal Medicine* 167(8):828–833.

Volandes, A. E., M. J. Barry, Y. Chang, and M. K. Paasche-Orlow. 2010. Improving decision making at the end of life with video images. *Medical Decision Making* 30(1):29–34.

Williams, M. V., D. W. Baker, E. G. Honig, T. M. Lee, and A. Nowlan. 1998. Inadequate literacy is a barrier to asthma knowledge and self-care. *Chest* 114(4):1008–1015.

Wolf, M. S., T. C. Davis, W. Shrank, D. N. Rapp, P. F. Bass, U. M. Connor, M. Clayman, and R. M. Parker. 2007. To err is human: Patient misinterpretations of prescription drug label instructions. *Patient Education and Counseling* 67(3):293–300.

Wolf, M. S., L. M. Curtis, K. Waite, S. C. Bailey, L. A. Hedlund, T. C. Davis, W. H. Shrank, R. M. Parker, and A. J. J. Wood. 2011a. Helping patients simplify and safely use complex prescription regimens. *Archives of Internal Medicine* 171(4):300–305.

Wolf, M. S., T. C. Davis, L. M. Curtis, J. A. Webb, S. C. Bailey, W. H. Shrank, L. Lindquist, B. Ruo, M. V. Bocchini, R. M. Parker, and A. J. J. Wood. 2011b. Effect of standardized, patient-centered label instructions to improve comprehension of prescription drug use. *Medical Care* 49(1):96–100.

Woolf, S. H., R. E. Glasgow, A. Krist, C. Bartz, S. A. Flocke, J. S. Holtrop, S. F. Rothemich, and E. R. Wald. 2005. Putting it together: Finding success in behavior change through integration of services. *Annals of Family Medicine* 3(Suppl 2):S20–S27.

Wynia, M. K., M. Johnson, T. P. McCoy, L. P. Griffin, and C. Y. Osborn. 2010. Validation of an organizational communication climate assessment toolkit. *American Journal of Medical Quality* 25(6):436–443.

Yin, H. S., B. P. Dreyer, G. Foltin, L. van Schaick, and A. L. Mendelsohn. 2007. Association of low caregiver health literacy with reported use of nonstandardized dosing instruments and lack of knowledge of weight-based dosing. *Ambulatory Pediatrics* 7(4):292–298.

Appendix B

Agenda

Institute of Medicine
Roundtable on Health Literacy

Attributes of a Health Literate Organization
Conference Center
20 F Street, NW
Washington, D.C.

November 16, 2011

WORKSHOP — Conference Rooms A & B

8:30–8:45	Welcome and Overview *George Isham, Chair*
8:45–9:05	Presentation of Commissioned Paper on Attributes of a Health Literate Organization *Dean Schillinger, M.D.* *Professor of Medicine in Residence* *Chief, Division of General Internal Medicine* *University of California at San Francisco*
9:05–9:30	Discussion

The first three panels will provide reactions to the commissioned paper from health care providers who practice in different kinds of health care organizations. Each presenter will be asked to respond to a set of questions.

9:30–10:30	PANEL 1 PRESENTATIONS AND DISCUSSION
9:30–9:45	Public Hospital System *Lauren Johnston* *Chief Nursing Officer and Senior Assistant Vice President* *Patient Centered Care* *New York City Health & Hospital Corporation*
9:45–10:00	Public Clinic *Debra Dever* *Chief Executive Officer* *Loudoun Community Health Center*
10:00–10:30	Discussion
10:30–10:50	**BREAK**
10:50–12:00	PANEL 2 PRESENTATIONS AND DISCUSSION
10:50–11:05	Private Practice *Isabel Hoverman, M.D.* *Austin Internal Medicine Associates, LLC*
11:05–11:20	Pharmacy Chain *Darren Townzen, R.Ph., M.B.A.* *Director of Health and Wellness Systems* *Wal-Mart*
11:20–12:00	Discussion
12:00–1:00	**LUNCH** Boardroom
1:00–2:00	PANEL 3 PRESENTATIONS AND DISCUSSION
1:00–1:15	Dental Practice *William Calnon, D.D.S.* *President, American Dental Association* *Private practice general dentistry*
1:15–1:30	Home Health *Cynthia Horton* *Visiting Nurses of El Paso*
1:30–2:00	Discussion

2:00–3:15 PANEL 4 PRESENTATIONS AND DISCUSSION

The final panel will provide reactions to the commissioned paper from individuals in various organizations that can or do provide incentives for organizational efforts in particular areas. Each panelist will be asked to respond to a set of questions.

2:00–2:15 Joint Commission
Ana Pujols-McKee, M.D.
Chief Medical Officer, Joint Commission Enterprise
Executive Vice President of Healthcare Improvement, The Joint Commission

2:15–2:30 Employer
John Neuberger
Director of Client Partnerships
Quad/Med, Quad Graphics

2:30–2:45 Centers for Medicare and Medicaid Services
Shari Ling, M.D.
Acting Deputy Chief Medical Officer

2:45–3:15 Discussion

3:15–3:45 Reflections on Lessons Learned

3:45 ADJOURN WORKSHOP

Appendix C

Speaker Biographical Sketches

William R. Calnon, D.D.S., who practices general dentistry in Rochester, New York, is president of the American Dental Association (ADA). Dr. Calnon's previous responsibilities with the ADA include serving as the 2nd district trustee to the board of trustees as well as a four-year term on the Council on Dental Practice. He is past president of the New York State Dental Association, the Seventh District Dental Society, and the Monroe County Dental Society. He served on the New York State Board of Dentistry and was an examiner for the Northeast Board of Dental Examiners. In addition, he is a fellow of the American College of Dentists, the International College of Dentists, and the Pierre Fauchard Academy. Dr. Calnon graduated magna cum laude from the State University of New York (SUNY) College of Environmental Science and Forestry at Syracuse University and received his dental degree from the SUNY at Buffalo School of Dental Medicine.

Debra Dever, chief executive officer of the Loudoun Community Health Center (LCHC), has over 35 years of experience in health care, with 15 years in executive positions in a variety of settings, including acute care, home health care, rehabilitation, and primary care. She has a master's degree in nursing service administration and a bachelor's degree in nursing. She has a multicultural background, including having lived in four foreign countries: Mexico, India, Spain, and Israel. Most recently, prior to coming to LCHC Ms. Dever was the executive director of Benewah Medical and Wellness Center, an award-winning tribally owned Federally

Qualified Health Center (FQHC) in Northern Idaho for 7 1/2 years. Ms. Dever was responsible for putting together LCHC from scratch. Since seeing its first patients in May 2007, LCHC has cared for over 10,000 patients and grown from a staff of 5 to a staff of 50.

Cynthia Horton has served as the director of development for the Visiting Nurse Association (VNA) of El Paso for the last 9 years. Her responsibilities include raising money, writing grants, and building awareness for charitable health care for those who are uninsured, underinsured, or indigent. She raises awareness and money for the medically homebound who, without these funds, would be unable to receive the care they need. VNA is the only not-for-profit home health care agency in El Paso and provides over $400,000 for charitable services each year.

Having been a foster parent for 17 years, she is still very involved in training and informal presentations regarding foster care, and she presents information to the community on a variety of topics. She volunteers with different organizations and serves on several local boards. Her community involvement includes the El Paso Center for Children and El Paso Families Project, the Habitat for Humanity board of directors, YWCA del Norte Region board member, the YWCA children's advisory committee, the Better Business Bureau board of directors, the Computer Career Center advisory board, and the Executive Forum, and she is a Women's Fund of El Paso Fortune 400 Member.

Isabel V. Hoverman, M.D., MACP, is a board-certified internist in private practice in Austin, Texas. She has served on the board of directors of the American College of Physicians Foundation, a health literacy organization, and the board of regents of the American College of Physicians. She is chair of the board of commissioners of The Joint Commission and a member of the board of directors of The Joint Commission International, organizations whose mission is to improve the quality and safety of health care in the United States and internationally through evaluation, accreditation, and education services. She is a member of the State Review Program Committee (SRPC) of the Texas Medical Foundation, the quality improvement organization for Texas that contracts with the Center for Medicare Services to improve the effectiveness, efficiency, and quality of services delivered to Medicare beneficiaries in Texas. The SRCP reviews patient complaints and meets with physicians and hospitals where quality or utilization problems have been identified in order to develop individual and systems-based approaches to correct and improve care at the physician and institutional level.

Dr. Hoverman helped establish the General Internal Medicine Statewide Preceptorship Program, which places first-year medical students from eight Texas medical schools in practicing internists' offices. She is a clinical assistant professor of medicine at the University of Texas Medical Branch at Galveston.

Debra Keller, M.D., M.P.H., is a graduate of Barnard College, received her medical degree from University of Pennsylvania School of Medicine, and completed her master's of public health at the Harvard School of Public Health, where she worked with Dr. Rima Rudd in the design of an educational module on health literacy for the Department of Veterans Affairs and carried out institutional assessments of the health literacy environments in public and private hospitals. She is currently a senior internal medicine resident in the San Francisco General Primary Care Program at University of California, San Francisco.

Shari Ling, M.D., serves as a medical officer in the Office of Clinical Standards at the Centers for Medicare and Medicaid Services (CMS) and is currently serving as the acting deputy chief medical officer. In addition to supporting the work of quality measurement nursing homes, home health agencies, End-Stage Renal Disease Network, and, more recently, the development of measures for new quality-reporting programs in inpatient rehabilitation facilities, long-term care acute hospitals, and hospices, she has also been the lead coordinator and facilitator of the monthly Office of Clinical Standards and Quality measures forum. Dr. Ling represents CMS on the U.S. Department of Health and Human Services (HHS) multiple chronic conditions workgroup and on the post-acute-care/long-term-care workgroup of the National Quality Forum's Measures Application Partnership. She also leads the measures and data sources sub-workgroup for the HHS Action Plan for HAI Prevention in Long-Term Care Facilities and leads the clinical sub-group for the National Alzheimer's Project Act.

Dr. Ling is a rheumatologist and geriatrician who received her medical training at Georgetown University School of Medicine, where she graduated as a member of the Alpha Omega Alpha Honor Society. She received her clinical training in internal medicine and rheumatology at Georgetown University Medical Center, followed by geriatric medicine at Johns Hopkins University. She remained on faculty at Johns Hopkins for 5 years, after which she worked for 8 years in the intramural research program of the National Institutes of Health in the National Institute on Aging as a staff clinician studying human aging and age-associated chronic diseases with attention to musculoskeletal conditions and mobility function. She continues to serve as a part-time faculty member in the Division of Geriatric Medicine and Gerontology at Johns Hopkins University School of Medicine and in the Division of Rheumatology, Allergy, and Clinical Immunology at the University of Maryland and enjoys seeing patients on a voluntary basis through the Veterans Administration Medical Center in Baltimore. She is a also a gerontologist who received her training in direct service from the Ethel Percy Andrus Gerontology Center at the University of Southern California, later serving as the codirector of the Andrus Older Adult Counseling Center.

John Neuberger is director of client partnerships at Quad/Graphics and is responsible for the contracting and ongoing relationships with all health care partners that serve the needs of Quad/Graphics' 20,000 employees throughout the United States.

Mr. Neuberger brings more than 35 years of health care experience to his position. Before assuming his current position, he served as vice president of operations of QuadMed for 8 years. This is a wholly owned subsidiary of Quad/Graphics that manages onsite clinics throughout the country. Mr. Neuberger had been with QuadMed for 15 years.

Prior to joining QuadMed, Mr. Neuberger served as regional vice president of physician integration with Covenant Healthcare for more than 7 years. He also served as president of Covenant Medical Group, an 82-physician multi-specialty group located in the Milwaukee area.

Mr. Neuberger received his bachelor's degree from St. Francis Seminary, Milwaukee, and his master's degree in health services administration from St. Francis University in Joliet, Illinois.

Ana Pujols-McKee, M.D., is the executive vice president and chief medical officer of The Joint Commission. In this role Dr. McKee represents The Joint Commission enterprise as she focuses on and develops policies and strategies for promoting patient safety and quality improvement in health care. Her responsibilities include providing support to The Joint Commission's Patient Safety Advisory Group; overseeing work related to the development of the Sentinel Event Policy, National Patient Safety Goals, and *Sentinel Event Alerts;* supervising the Sentinel Event Database; and overseeing the functions of the Standards Interpretation Group and the Office of Quality Monitoring. Dr. McKee also provides clinical guidance and support to the Joint Commission Center for Transforming Healthcare, Joint Commission Resources, and Joint Commission International.

Prior to her current position, Dr. McKee served as the chief medical officer and associate executive director at Penn Presbyterian Medical Center, University of Pennsylvania Health System, and as a clinical associate professor of medicine at the University of Pennsylvania School of Medicine. She also served as the medical director for the Philadelphia Health Department's freestanding health centers.

Dr. McKee is a former board member of the American Cancer Society, the Pennsylvania Health Care Cost Containment Council, Health Partners

Philadelphia, and Philadelphia AIDS Consortium and is the former board chair for the Pennsylvania Safety Authority and vice chair for the Public Health Management Corporation. Dr. McKee also sits on the board of Quality Insights of Pennsylvania. In addition, she served on the Food and Drug Administration's advisory committee and on several committees of the National Institutes of Health.

Dr. McKee holds a bachelor's degree in psychology from the State University of New York at Binghamton and a medical degree from Hahnemann Medical College and Hospital in Philadelphia. She completed her residency at Presbyterian Medical Center in Philadelphia and is board certified in internal medicine. Dr. McKee participated as an affiliate member of the Robert Wood Johnson Clinical Scholars Program and concentrated her studies in health care administration in a nondegree program at the Wharton School.

Dean Schillinger, M.D., is professor of medicine in residence at the University of California, San Francisco (UCSF), and chief of the UCSF division of general internal medicine at San Francisco General Hospital (SFGH). He is a practicing primary care physician at SFGH, an urban public hospital, where he sees patients, teaches in the primary care residency program, and conducts research. In his prior administrative roles, he has directed the Medi-Cal managed care clinic at SFGH and the general medicine clinic at SFGH and has been the director of clinical operations for the Department of Medicine. Dr. Schillinger also serves as chief of the Diabetes Prevention and Control Program for the California Department of Public Health.

Author of over 130 scientific manuscripts, Dr. Schillinger carries out research related to health care for vulnerable populations and is an internationally recognized expert in health communication science. His work focuses on literacy, health communication, and chronic disease prevention and management. He has carried out a number of studies exploring the impact of limited health literacy on the care of patients with diabetes and heart disease and has developed and evaluated communication programs tailored to the literacy and language needs of patients with chronic disease. He has been the recipient of research grants from the National Institutes of Health, the Agency for Healthcare Research and Quality, the U.S. Centers for Disease Control and Prevention, the California Endowment, the Commonwealth Fund, and the California Health Care Foundation. He has been honored with the 2003 Institute for Healthcare Advancement Research Award, the 2008 Research Award in Safety and Quality from the National Patient Safety Foundation, the 2009 Engel Award in Health Communication Research, and the California Association of Public Hospital Quality Leaders Award for this work. He was a coinvestigator for the

National Association of Public Health and Hospital Institute's Diabetes Quality Improvement Consortium.

Dr. Schillinger is the founding director of the UCSF Center for Vulnerable Populations (CVP), whose mission is to carry out innovative research to prevent and treat chronic disease in populations for whom social conditions often conspire to both promote chronic disease and make its management more challenging. CVP is based within the UCSF's department of medicine, located on the campus of San Francisco General Hospital and Trauma Center, the public health hospital of the city and county of San Francisco. CVP has distinguished itself as a practice-based research center whose work has helped translate research into community and public health practice as well as to infuse local practice back into research. CVP faculty members have coordinated eight randomized trials in community settings. Beyond the local communities it serves, CVP is nationally and internationally known for its research in health communication and health policy to reduce health disparities, with special expertise in the social determinants of health, including literacy, food policy, poverty, and minority status, as well as with a focus on the clinical conditions of prediabetes, diabetes, and cardiovascular disease, including hypertension, chronic kidney disease and heart failure. Dr. Schillinger currently directs the CVP health communications program.

In his capacity as chief of the Diabetes Prevention and Control Program for the California Department of Public Health, he has been expanding the program's work in health communications, social and environmental determinants of diabetes, and health disparities. In this capacity he has partnered with Youth Speaks, a youth empowerment organization that harnesses social media, to advance a California diabetes prevention initiative. Dr. Schillinger is also principal investigator, along with the Kaiser Division of Research, for the UCSF component of a P30 Center for Type 2 Diabetes Translational Research recently funded by the National Institute of Diabetes and Digestive and Kidney Diseases.

Dr. Schillinger has a strong commitment and outstanding track record of training fellows and junior faculty and has been the primary or secondary mentor for 10 K level career development award recipients. He was awarded the 2010 Outstanding Bay Area Clinical Research Mentor Prize by the UCSF Clinical and Translational Sciences Institute, the Kaiser Division of Research, the Palo Alto Medical Foundation Research Institute, and Genentech. He was the first health communication scientist to receive this award. Dr. Schillinger contributed to the 2004 Institute of Medicine report on health literacy, is a section editor for the textbooks *Understanding Health Literacy* (AMA press) and *Caring for Vulnerable and Underserved Populations* (Lange series/McGraw Hill, 2007), is a member of the American College of Physicians' health communication advisory board, and serves on the editorial board of the journal *Patient Education and Counseling*. In 2000 he completed an Open Society Institute Advocacy Fellowship working with California Literacy, Inc., a nonprofit educational organization that helps people gain literacy skills, to advance the California Health Literacy Initiative. With respect to chronic disease control on the global level, he recently returned from a semester as visiting scholar at the University of Chile's School of Public Health to help develop chronic disease prevention and treatment initiatives and has served as a consultant to the National Health Group in Singapore and the Scotland Department of Health on chronic disease and health promotion initiatives.

Darren Townzen is currently the director of health and wellness systems for Wal-Mart Stores, Inc. In 1988 he received a bachelor of science degree from the Southwestern Oklahoma State University School of Pharmacy, and in 2006 he earned a masters of business administration from Webster University. In 1989 he started work for the Wal-Mart Stores pharmacy division as a pharmacist in east Texas before coming into the general office in 1995 for other responsibilities. Current responsibilities include prescription insurance connectivity, billing standards, prescription monitoring programs, and electronic prescribing. He has been a member of the National Council for Prescription Drug Programs since 2005 and is active in Work Group 2 Product Identification and Work Group 9 Government Programs, where he is currently serving in the role as a standardization cochair and a member of the board of trustees.

Ross Wilson, M.D., is senior vice president and chief medical officer at the New York City Health and Hospital Corporation. As chief medical officer at the New York City Health and Hospital Corporation, Dr. Wilson has oversight of clinical care delivery at 11 teaching hospitals, 6 diagnostic and treatment centers, 80 community clinics, and 4 long-term care facilities which provide care to more than 1.3 million patients annually. The system also includes the MetroPlus health plan and a home care service. Prior to taking on this role at the largest municipal public health system in the United States, Dr. Wilson was the director of the Centre for Healthcare Improvement in the Northern Sydney Central Coast Health Service in Australia. In addition he has had many leadership, board, and management roles in Australian and international public health systems.

Dr. Wilson was the chairman of the strategic advisory board for the International Forum for Quality and Safety in Health Care and international advisor to the Australian Commission for Safety and Quality in Health Care until July 2009. As leader of the Quality in Australian Health Care Study (1993–1995) and, more recently, the Eastern Mediterranean and African regional study of patient safety in developing economies for the World Health Organization (WHO) from 2005 to 2008, Dr. Wilson has a long research and publication experience in the epidemiology of patient safety. Since 1999 his key interests have been leadership, training, and project support for clinical improvement through the Clinical Practice Improvement program and its associated projects.

At a strategic level, Dr. Wilson has been a member of the WHO World Alliance for Patient Safety Expert Advisory Group, a contributor to the WHO Patient Safety Research Council, a member of the WHO International Steering Committee for Patient Safety Solutions, a member of the Asia–Pacific Regional Council for Joint Commission International, and a member of the editorial board of the *British Medical Journal*.

Until 2005 Dr. Wilson had a clinical role as senior specialist in intensive care medicine at Royal North Shore Hospital, a teaching hospital of the University of Sydney.